Understanding Medical Information

A User's Guide to Informatics and Decision Making

Notice

Medicine is an ever-changing science. As new research and clinical experience broaden our knowledge, changes in treatment and drug therapy are required. The author and the publisher of this work have checked with sources believed to be reliable in their efforts to provide information that is complete and generally in accord with the standards accepted at the time of publication. However, in view of the possibility of human error or changes in medical sciences, neither the author nor the publisher nor any other party who has been involved in the preparation or publication of this work warrants that the information contained herein is in every respect accurate or complete, and they disclaim all responsibility for any errors or omissions or for the results obtained from use of the information contained in this work. Readers are encouraged to confirm the information contained herein with other sources. For example and in particular, readers are advised to check the product information sheet included in the package of each drug they plan to administer to be certain that the information contained in this work is accurate and that changes have not been made in the recommended dose or in the contraindications for administration. This recommendation is of particular importance in connection with new or infrequently used drugs.

UNDERSTANDING MEDICAL INFORMATION

A User's Guide to Informatics and Decision Making

Theresa J. Jordan, MA, PhD

Associate Professor and Chair
Department of Applied Psychology
New York University, School of Education
New York, New York
Medical Informatics Specialist
Department of Medicine and National Tuberculosis Center
New Jersey Medical School
University of Medicine and Dentistry of New Jersey
Newark, New Jersey

McGraw-Hill
Medical Publishing Division

New York   Chicago   San Francisco   Lisbon   London   Madrid   Mexico City
Milan   New Delhi   San Juan   Seoul   Singapore   Sydney   Toronto

McGraw-Hill

A Division of The McGraw·Hill Companies

Understanding Medical Information: A User's Guide to Informatics and Decision Making

1234567890 DOC DOC 0987654321

ISBN 0–8385–9272–4

This book was set in Korinna Roman by Pine Tree Composition.
The editors were Shelley Reinhardt and Karen Davis.
The production supervisor was Catherine Saggese.
The cover designer was Mary McDonnell
The index was prepared by Angie Wiley.
R. R. Donnelley, Crawfordsville, was printer and binder.

This book is printed on acid-free paper.

Library of Congress Cataloging-in-Publication Data

Jordan, Theresa J.
   Understanding medical information/Theresa J. Jordan.
     p.; cm.
   Includes bibliographical references and index.
   ISBN 0-8385-9272-4 (pbk.)
    1. Medical informatics. I. Title.
    [DNLM: 1. Medical Informatics. W 26.5 J82u2001]
   R858 .J67 2001
   610--dc21   2001030566

For my mother,
Helen J. Balazs,
who gave me, among so much else,
the gift of her fascination with the medical world

Contents

PREFACE

To understand medical information in today's world, it is necessary to have a grasp of very diverse and divergent realms of knowledge that extend beyond clinical knowledge of diseases and their treatments. The study of medical information is not yet a clearly defined field, although programs of study in medical "informatics" have been emerging in medical schools and other health and technology oriented disciplines. The purpose of this book is to gather together under one cover, perhaps for the first time, the most important components necessary for understanding medical information, so that readers might find a door into a rather elusive "meta-field" that crosses many disciplines and borrows many sophisticated tools.

The explosion of information in medicine that has been occurring for the past few decades has exerted pressures both on information management technologies and on the practice of medicine, including the development of medical and public health policies. Because more information exists than ever before in medical fields, clinicians and policymakers are called upon increasingly to base their decisions on "evidence" presented in a formally analyzed manner—and to move away from reliance on anecdotal records or personal experience. One result of the information explosion is the increasing pressure for what is called "evidence-based medicine." In order to make clinical decisions, public health policies, or individual choices that qualify as "evidence based" it is essential for contemporary professionals to be able both to access and to understand medical information.

The audience of *Understanding Medical Information: A User's Guide to Informatics and Decision Making* includes students of medicine, nursing, and the health-related professions who seek a short, reliable guide to tapping into, and understanding, today's vast reservoir of medical information. Clinicians can use the book as a refresher.

Lay consumers of medical information who, for a variety of reasons, wish to better understand medical reports, journal articles, and the contours of modern medicine will also enjoy reading this lively and instructive book.

This book sets the stage for understanding medical information in Chapters 1 and 2, which explain how it is that we have arrived at an incredible level of technological sophistication, a wealth of knowledge at our fingertips, a demand for evidence-based decisions and policies, and the problem of so much uncertainty. Chapter 3 provides an overview of types of medical research, the role of statistics in evaluating studies, and the social and ethical issues that impact dramatically on the research that is done as well as what is not funded, not approved, or not published. Chapters 4, 5, and 6 comprise a central core of knowledge about the high- as well as lower-tech processes by which we make diagnoses of individual patients, assess the health of populations, make decisions about treatments under conditions of uncertainty, and attempt to provide the best prognostic judgments possible given the great complexity and diversity among patients. The final sections of the book, Chapters 7 and 8, provide conceptual as well as practical guidelines for assessing the quality of medical information available on the Internet, explain the ways in which Internet resources might best be used to capture good information, and confront the current realities of what can and cannot be expected from "artificial intelligence."

This book is not intended to serve the role of a traditional research design text, a how-to manual for computer applications, or a comprehensive user's guide to the Internet. However, it addresses issues in all these areas—and then some—to the extent that they bear on the needs of today's consumers of medical information. It is intended for use either as a primary or ancillary text in both preprofessional and continuing education courses, as well as a resource for anyone who seeks to be equipped better with the concepts that make medical information more accessible and digestible.

Hopefully, this book will be used in a diversity of ways by a range of individuals who are seeking a guide to the expanding frontiers made possible by revolutionary strides in data management and communications technologies and by the related explosions in medical/health care research.

ACKNOWLEDGMENTS

Thank you to all my students, past and present, in clinical medicine and in psychology—you have been my most important teachers. You led me to the areas that you found confusing and engaged me in the dialogues that initiated the idea for this book. Your feedback on my teaching enabled me to refine, expand, and clarify my approaches, my examples, and my organization in ways that best suited the needs of a broad audience.

Thank you to the universities that nurtured and appreciated my explorations in medical informatics. The Department of Medicine, the New Jersey Medical School National Tuberculosis Center, and the Sammy Davis Jr. National Liver Institute, all at the University of Medicine and Dentistry of New Jersey, have been instrumental in shaping my career in medical informatics. Dr. Lee B. Reichman at the National Tuberculosis Center continues to provide support and encouragement for my research and other writings in the area of clinical decision analysis. New York University's School of Education and, in particular, the Department of Applied Psychology, have welcomed openly work in an area not traditionally encompassed by psychology. New York University has provided a climate in which I am able to pursue diverse goals with the gift of academic freedom.

Books can grow in mysterious ways. Dr. Justin Graham at Stanford University never planned to be part of *Understanding Medical Information*. However, his review of the draft manuscript elegantly provided simple insights that prompted me to reframe and rewrite an entire chapter. To Dr. Graham, thank you for your generosity and the unanticipated yet essential contributions to this work.

To my husband, Richard L. Montgomery, DDS, MPH: Your input throughout this book, your critical readings, and especially your assistance with the chapters on public health and on Internet-based information have been invaluable. Without your constant, loving support, your intellectual contributions, and your unfailing help in keeping day-to-day life on track, this book could not have been written.

To my young daughter, Tui Jordan: So many times you stood at the door of my study as I worked at the computer and asked, "Mama, are you done yet?" And when I said no, you smiled anyway, and threw me a kiss. Your smiles and your love are the sweetness that remind me always what a blessing it is to be your mother.

To my mom, Helen J. Balazs, to whom this book is dedicated: As long as I can remember, you modeled an approach to the medical world that taught me to approach it without fear and with great wonder. You talked with me about anything and everything and valued my questions. You could have been an incredible physician. You are, and have been, an incredible mother. Thank you.

Finally, to my editors: Cheryl Mehalik at Appleton & Lange nurtured this project in its initial stages, and stood by it through many of my life's challenges. I appreciate sincerely your interest and support. Shelley Reinhardt at McGraw-Hill picked up where the midwife left off, and enthusiastically helped me as the project grew into a finished book. And, at the end, Karen Davis at McGraw-Hill provided the wonderful, close collaboration essential in the final stages of production. I needed all of you—many thanks.

Theresa J. Jordan

New York, New York
September 2001

1

Chapter One

The Continuing Revolution in Medicine

. . . Science had become the key to health and illness, and patients theoretically could master some of this science, and then take responsibility for helping the doctor fight or manage the illness. The doctor would be in part a teacher of human biology, and indeed would try to dispel mystery, not cultivate it.

At least in theory. In reality mystery remains, but it has a different location: it lives on the frontier of technology. Computed tomography, magnetic resonance imaging, laser surgery, laparoscopy, television-assisted microsurgery, lithotripsy, radioactive isotope tracing, radiotherapy—these are only a few of the state-of-the-art methods that doctors love and patients increasingly demand. These methods often work, but they cost a great deal of money, and they are certainly not always cost-effective. However, they do pretty much guarantee mystery-in fact, the way they work is usually beyond the technological grasp of the doctors who make use of them. Only some engineers and physicists understand them. Doctor and patient stand together, grateful and humbled, before what almost seem to be technological gods.

Melvin J. Konner

Introduction...

■INFORMATION, INFORMATICS AND EVIDENCE-BASED MEDICINE

Since the early 1980s, medicine has been undergoing a continuing revolution, the essence of which is best captured by the term "informatics." **Informatics** may be thought of as a meta-field because it involves concepts and tools from many disciplines, including statistics and biostatistics, research design, computer programming, database management, and mathematical modeling. The tools of informatics are used for the purposes of generating, organizing, and making accessible and intelligible huge amounts of information. Medical informatics is the application of informatics tools and purposes to medical information.

An explosion of medical information has occurred during the past few decades, an explosion that has coincided with the invention of new medical tools, particularly for diagnosis. The information generated by scientific studies and by the application of new diagnostic and treatment modalities created, in turn, a pressing need for techniques and technologies that could manage masses of medical data. New methods for gathering, storing, retrieving, analyzing, and interpreting information became essential in order to "capture" medical information and to make it available quickly for use by practitioners, policymakers, and patients.

Simultaneously, and rather independently, engineers were developing the computer technologies that could meet such needs. Beginning with the advent of the high speed microcomputer up through today's instant access to literally a world of material on the Internet, information is accessible on virtually any topic.

The availability of new computer technologies and the concurrent emergence of massive amounts of medical information provided a fertile environment for the development of "evidence-based medicine," a conceptual framework for clinical decisions that has its origins in work done at McMaster

Medical School during the 1980s. Evidence-based medicine may be understood as one important application of medical informatics. In evidence-based medicine, the clinician makes medical decisions through a process of searching medical literature, evaluating the quality of information available on a particular topic, and using what has been found and judged to be sound in the everyday practice of clinical medicine. Evidence-based medicine is a product of both the information explosion in medicine and the development of sophisticated computer technologies, since it is based on the assumptions that "evidence" exists and can be found.

Another critical aspect of the continuing revolution in medicine is the unprecedented availability of medical information to the general public through personal computing and Internet access. Patients can communicate, retrieve, and exchange information at a level of sophistication that has never before occurred.

With high speed computing, networking capabilities, massive amounts of medical information available to health care providers and consumers alike, and medical practices requiring the retrieval and use of information on a broad scale, medicine has been able to enter fully the "information age." In less than a century, it has leapt from the bedside to the computer. This leap is the hallmark of the informatics revolution in medicine.

■AN EMBARRASSMENT OF RICHES

The boon in medical knowledge contributes unprecedented benefits to health care, but also creates problems—the kinds of problems that arise from trying to keep pace with an ever-shifting, self-correcting, and ever-escalating body of information.

In response, medicine has become extraordinarily mathematical and computerized. And the math and computer "tools" that have been developed to manage medical information are not necessarily extensions of traditional mathematics or computer programming. Consequently, yesterday's math whiz might find herself lost in the new worlds of mathematical modeling with decision analysis, artificial intelligence, and uncertainty. Small wars have been fought among medical informatics specialists over the use of techniques most professionals have never encountered, e.g., the question of whether rule-based systems are preferable to pattern recognition approaches for making computer-generated diagnoses.

Medical journals that once were replete with reports of single, interesting cases, now abound with multicenter trials, meta-analyses, decision analyses, multidimensional sensitivity analyses, Markov models, Cox regressions, and a myriad of other sophisticated approaches to the solution of our health problems. It has become impossible for many individuals—physicians, other health care providers, and health care consumers—to understand both the statistical and the clinical or biochemical aspects of today's reports of medical research.

On the other hand, neglecting to familiarize oneself with the fundamental concepts of medical informatics means surrendering to an irresponsible default option: uncritical acceptance of the few intelligible conclusions articulated in the abstract of a scholarly journal or, worse, the overly simplified ruminations of the popular media. The result of this neglect is a growing medical illiteracy across nearly all segments of the population. Patients have great difficulty comprehending the complex trade-offs inherent in medical decisions; nonphysician health care providers experience increased difficulty reading both medical literature and physician reports; and physicians themselves express frustration with "incomprehensible" informatics techniques published in their own fields.

Another skill that has become essential for a broad range of health care providers and allied health professionals is an ability to "surf the Web" to find answers to medical questions. This means that an increasingly higher degree of computer literacy is needed, extending beyond the isolated desktop computer to complex communications networks. It also means that health care providers must cope often with data in forms other than the typical journal article or textbook. Information available on the Internet/World Wide Web may be in the form of databases not yet or only partially analyzed, and preliminary reports or commentaries that have not been peer reviewed for quality control. Consequently, the new technologies require the user to have sharper skills in both computer technology and critical analysis of research, as protection against "misinformation."

A critical point that must be kept in mind while delving into the wealth of information available even to the casual user, is that **information does not necessarily equal knowledge, wisdom, or truth.** More than ever before, it has become the responsibility of the user to determine the quality of medical information. We have entered into a kind of contract in which we, the users, gain access to massive amounts of information—in return for which we bear the responsibility of evaluating the information critically and ethically, and in doing so take on the burden that belonged traditionally to the peer reviewers of medical journals.

■KEEPING UP WITH THE REVOLUTION

Attempting to keep pace with the informatics revolution is an awesome task. However, "keeping pace" can mean a number of things. It can mean understanding the engineering details of the newest computer on the market, or the physics that permits high-tech magnetic resonance imaging. On the other hand, it can mean developing a basic understanding of what some of the new techniques are intended to accomplish as well as how to "read" the results. For most health care providers, the latter kind of understanding is sufficient. In fact, it is an admirable feat of continuing education! It is certainly possible to read critically the results of a decision analysis without knowing how the computer program that generated it arrived at a mathematical maximization of life expectancy, or to consider the output from an artificially intelligent diagnostic program without knowing how computerized frames were used to work toward pattern recognition.

As medical information and the technology to manage it continue to grow, the task of mastering every detail becomes increasingly impossible. One must select for study those aspects of informatics that are particularly essential to one's own field or interests, bearing in mind that every area will require updating on a regular basis.

As you sample the materials presented in this book, perhaps your appetite will be whetted to pursue some topics in more detail than others. References are provided as a guide for further learning. On the other hand, be cautious about venturing too far afield from your goals, lest you find yourself mired in some mysteries of physics or engineering that may be of little interest or use to you. The last section of this chapter provides guidelines for developing a practical and possible level of informatics literacy. Approach it with this maxim in mind, *"Keep far from me the delusion that I can accomplish all things"* (Maimonides—twelfth century physician's prayer).

A Glimpse of History

Toward the end of the twentieth century, educators began to realize that advances in information technologies had begun to outpace our ability to train future physicians in these techniques (Rootenberg, 1992). As medical schools attempt desperately to enter the information age, the wealth of medical knowledge to be imparted leaves even less space in the medical curriculum to educate physicians and other health care providers in the techniques designed to manage and analyze this knowledge. It seems there is both too much information and too much technology. Yet, to make progress in health care, it seems that there must be more of both in professional school curricula as well as in continuing education.

Why look to history when we are overwhelmed by what is happening *now?* Perhaps an historical perspective will help relieve some of the panic that arises when individuals see themselves "left out of" or "left behind in" the informatics revolution. In the full timeframe of medicine, whose beginning can be set in the Paleolithic period (c. 30,000 B.C.), the intrusion of the informatics revolution has occurred in the last .0625% of medical history. Feeling left out or left behind is typical when something so new happens so quickly, and impacts so widely and dramatically (Figure 1a).

■CLINICAL VERSUS RESEARCH MEDICINE

Much of the practice of medicine in contemporary U.S. hospitals finds its roots somewhere in the tradition that William Osler brought to Johns Hopkins University Hospital. At the turn of the nineteenth century, Osler's proclamation that the practice of medicine should be wedded to science found wide support among physicians. Osler insisted that hospitals serve as laboratories in which disease and treatment could be observed and studied intensively. It is from Osler that we have inherited many hospital routines that persist in some form to this day. For example, medical students are called "clerks" and their rotations through the clinical curriculum "clerkships." This language is based on Osler's notion that students act somewhat as clerks in that they should be responsible for collecting rigorous information regarding their patients. Bedside rounds, or "morning report," is an Osler legacy, during which medical students report on their cases to other students and senior medical faculty. Osler initiated the term "resident" when he insisted that house officers remain overnight in their hospitals to immerse themselves fully in the environment of disease.

Osler's insistence that medicine be wedded to science, and that voluminous information be collected on each patient, were first steps toward an information explosion in medicine. Without the impetus to collect clinical data, and to subject it to scientific study, it is unlikely that the same path to an informatics revolution would have occurred.

On the other hand, Osler's insistence on bedside rounds as the primary teaching tool as well as the embodiment of a marriage between medical practice and science proved problematic. The "science" of medicine had made little progress at Osler's time. Little was known about the causes of many dis-

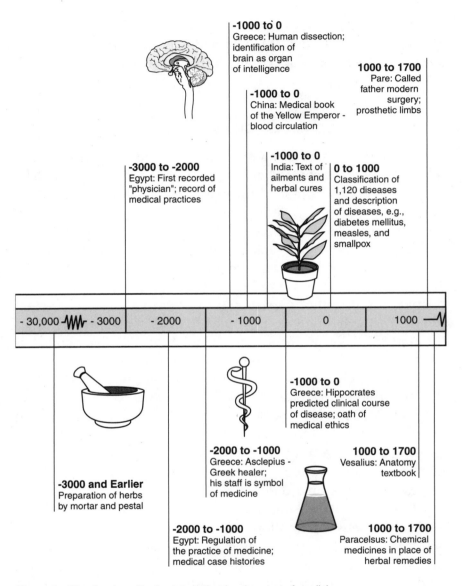

-1000 to 0
Greece: Human dissection;
identification of
brain as organ
of intelligence

-1000 to 0
China: Medical book
of the Yellow Emperor -
blood circulation

1000 to 1700
Pare: Called
father modern
surgery;
prosthetic limbs

-3000 to -2000
Egypt: First recorded
"physician"; record of
medical practices

-1000 to 0
India: Text of
ailments and
herbal cures

0 to 1000
Classification of
1,120 diseases
and description
of diseases, e.g.,
diabetes mellitus,
measles, and
smallpox

- 30,000 -ᴡᴡ- 3000   - 2000   - 1000   0   1000 -ᴧ-

-1000 to 0
Greece: Hippocrates
predicted clinical course
of disease; oath of
medical ethics

-2000 to -1000
Greece: Asclepius -
Greek healer;
his staff is symbol
of medicine

1000 to 1700
Vesalius: Anatomy
textbook

-3000 and Earlier
Preparation of herbs
by mortar and pestal

-2000 to -1000
Egypt: Regulation of
the practice of medicine;
medical case histories

1000 to 1700
Paracelsus: Chemical
medicines in place of
herbal remedies

Figure 1a Timeline for critical points in the development of medicine.

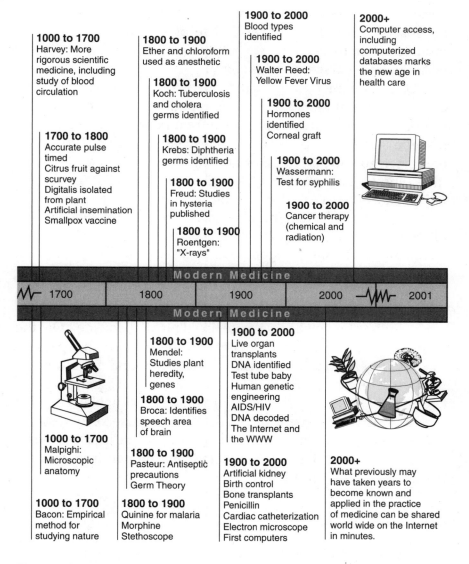

1900 to 2000
Blood types
identified

2000+
Computer access,
including
computerized
databases marks
the new age in
health care

1000 to 1700
Harvey: More
rigorous scientific
medicine, including
study of blood
circulation

1800 to 1900
Ether and chloroform
used as anesthetic

1900 to 2000
Walter Reed:
Yellow Fever Virus

1800 to 1900
Koch: Tuberculosis
and cholera
germs identified

1900 to 2000
Hormones
identified
Corneal graft

1700 to 1800
Accurate pulse
timed
Citrus fruit against
scurvey
Digitalis isolated
from plant
Artificial insemination
Smallpox vaccine

1800 to 1900
Krebs: Diphtheria
germs identified

1900 to 2000
Wassermann:
Test for syphilis

1800 to 1900
Freud: Studies
in hysteria
published

1900 to 2000
Cancer therapy
(chemical and
radiation)

1800 to 1900
Roentgen:
"X-rays"

Modern Medicine

–∿– 1700   1800   1900   2000 –∿∿– 2001

Modern Medicine

1800 to 1900
Mendel:
Studies plant
heredity,
genes

1900 to 2000
Live organ
transplants
DNA identified
Test tube baby
Human genetic
engineering
AIDS/HIV
DNA decoded
The Internet and
the WWW

1800 to 1900
Broca: Identifies
speech area
of brain

1000 to 1700
Malpighi:
Microscopic
anatomy

1800 to 1900
Pasteur: Antiseptic
precautions
Germ Theory

1900 to 2000
Artificial kidney
Birth control
Bone transplants
Penicillin
Cardiac catheterization
Electron microscope
First computers

2000+
What previously may
have taken years to
become known and
applied in the practice
of medicine can be shared
world wide on the Internet
in minutes.

1000 to 1700
Bacon: Empirical
method for
studying nature

1800 to 1900
Quinine for malaria
Morphine
Stethoscope

Figure 1a (continued)

eases, and far less about curing them. What was more likely to be observed was the clinical course of a disease once it had progressed to a level of severity requiring hospitalization—a rather narrow perspective for study.

Osler's impact took hold long before the advent of true clinical trial methodology, in which patients are randomly assigned to differing treatments, or a treatment versus nothing (a placebo), and both patient and physician are "blind" to whom has received which course of action. In the absence of clinical trials, the causes of various health outcomes were extremely difficult to determine. (On the other hand, the ethics of such "experimentation" remains a troublesome matter, and is discussed later in Chapter 3.)

In short, the Osler legacy has been a double-edged sword: It encouraged the conscientious collection and scrutiny of data from hospitalized patients, based on the notion that such data could provide a source of scientific knowledge. Thus, it provided impulsion toward science in clinical medicine. On the other hand, it provided a model of bedside learning that persists today, a model that is increasingly inefficient and not always in the best interests of the student since it limits his/her perspective to the kinds of diseases common at a particular site. For example, it is extremely unusual to see a case of malaria at University Hospital in Newark, New Jersey, but it is extremely common to treat individuals infected with human immunodeficiency virus (HIV) at that site.

■SUBSPECIALTIES

While Osler's educational legacy persists in many if not most teaching hospitals, at least one major departure from his dictums has occurred. Today's medical students spend a great deal of time studying with specialists and subspecialists, whose areas of expertise are increasingly specific and delimited.

Subspecialty training is, in fact, one response to the information explosion. If an individual cannot be expected to learn everything there is to learn in medicine, then it appears reasonable to encourage individuals to subspecialize in specific areas in which they can become exceedingly expert. For many years, medicine has consisted of specialties. Medical students typically decide among internal medicine, surgery, psychiatry, obstetrics/gynecology, pediatrics, orthopedics, etc., for post–graduate training. Subspecialties divide these areas even further into the study of particular organ systems or even single organs or appendages, e.g., the division of internal medicine into cardiology, gastroenterology, hepatology, oncology, hematology, endocrinology, rheumatology, renal disease, dermatology, allergy, and immunology.

The pendulum swings back and forth on the benefits and drawbacks of subspecialization, particularly since subspecialization can be at odds with holistic approaches to health care and a renewed interest in "family practice." Patients may wonder how their physicians can understand the impact of hand surgery on their whole lives, when their physicians read journals such as *Journal of the British Society for Surgery of the Hand,* which seems to isolate the hand from the rest of the human. However, it is clear now that one individual cannot be expected to learn everything there is to learn even within a subspecialty area. Due to several factors, including issues of insurance coverage for medical care, many patients use a combination of a primary physician (perhaps someone trained in family practice), as well as specialists (e.g., cardiologists) and subspecialists (e.g., cardiac surgeons) if and when specific needs arise.

■EDUCATIONAL CHANGE

We have been late in coming to terms with the dilemmas of contemporary medicine. For nearly 75 years, the "Flexner report" (Flexner, 1910), which was highly critical of much medical education in the United States at its time, shaped the teaching of medicine in this country and helped draw funds to institutions with first-rate faculty. This report emphasized the educational benefit of bedside "rounds" during which students could learn from expert physicians, such as William Osler, as they conducted face-to-face encounters with patients. Much learning was anecdotal, in that novice physicians would learn to make a diagnosis or decide on a treatment regimen because they recalled studying a patient during rounds who exemplified the particular medical problem.

However, in an era of scientific revolution, experience gleaned from yesterday's experts (though scientific at the time) may prove anachronistic tomorrow. For instance, what might have been a straightforward case of treatable pulmonary tuberculosis 10 years ago, may now be a deadly case of multiple drug-resistant tuberculosis in a patient with HIV disease. The range of diagnosable diseases and treatment options facing today's doctors will not be encountered during teaching rounds in hospitals with even the most diverse patient populations. And what once was considered a wise treatment choice or optimal diagnostic modality is likely to have been replaced several times over before today's students in various health care professions embark on their own careers.

In 1984, a document intruded on medical education which mandated that medical schools bring their educational practices into the information age. This document, *Physicians for the Twenty-First Century* (Panel on the General Professional Education of the Physician and College Preparation for Medicine, 1984), focused on enhancing the roles of computer-assisted diagnosis and treatment, as well as augmenting the role of informatics in clinical medicine. Above all, the document called for implementing high-technology medicine through the introduction of computer-based technologies into medical education.

Following in this direction, the Association of Physician Assistant Programs prepared their own report on *Physician Assistants for the Future* (1989), which called for statistics courses in physician-assistant programs, goals of enhanced problem-solving abilities, and skills in collecting and synthesizing data.

In 1993, the National Center for Nursing Research (now known as the National Institute for Nursing Research) published an agenda which addressed nursing informatics research, including the development of clinical databases, the design of information systems based on local needs, development of nursing workstations linked to integrated information systems, and methods for evaluating informatics goals.

Dentistry on the whole has been less direct in its call for informatics. However, a report on *Dental Education at the Cross-roads* (1995) conducted by the Institute of Medicine called for forging closer links between medicine and dentistry, transfer of technology across these health fields, and improved research. Articulation of these goals was intended as a first step toward bringing informatics more strongly into the forefront of dentistry.

While each of the above has been called an "agenda" for a field, they are nevertheless "position statements" that carry no weight unless they are supported financially and organizationally. Informatics sophistication requires an infrastructure to support information management and communication plus training plans that teach the techniques needed to make use of the infrastructure. As a result, fully implemented educational programs have lagged behind technological advances.

In the 1994 *Yearbook of Medical Informatics* (International Medical Informatics Association, 1994), several medical informatics training programs were described in detail: programs at Harvard University, University of Utah, and University of Heidelberg. These programs are well-refined, working prototypes of both predoctoral and postdoctoral training. Today, many other medical schools, as well as schools equipped to train physician assistants, dentists, nurses, and mental health specialists have adopted at least some aspects of informatics training.

■RIGHT AND WRONG

What might be confusing from the preceding section on medical history is that what appears at one time to be the correct course of treatment, or even the best educational strategy, might not, in fact, turn out to be the most correct or the best in the long run. This raises the often unmentionable issue: **That medicine is fallible.**

Many medical decisions are made on the basis of subjective values, incorrectly interpreted data, and misguided attempts to draw conclusions from scientific observations. Consider, for example, the early treatment of malaria. By the eighteenth century, the observation had been made repeatedly that malaria (which actually means "bad air") was associated with swamps. The conclusion drawn from this "scientific" observation is that bad air caused the disease and that it could be treated with "good air." Some conceptualizations of good air consisted of hanging a block of ice above the fever-ridden patient and fanning the cold air on his/her exposed body, a practice that killed more than it spared. The successful use of quinine to treat malaria did not emerge until the beginning of the nineteenth century. In spite of quinine's success, malaria continued to be treated for many years with bizarre and dangerous remedies, such as arsenic. Should that example seem too ancient to be realistic, consider the use of diethylstilbestrol to prevent miscarriage in millions of pregnant woman during the middle of the twentieth century. As the daughters of these women entered their reproductive years, some developed an otherwise rare and deadly cancer of the vagina. The sons of these women may be at increased risk for testicular cancer. Thus, a treatment that had appeared "good" in terms of the ability to prevent miscarriage, exhibited devastating effects a generation later.

It is difficult for many scientists, practitioners, and patients to accept the fact that medicine is a probabalistic rather than an exact science, that medical reasoning is often "fuzzy" (see Chapter 2), and that many errors are made along the road that is often mislabeled the road to progress. **Just as errors have been made in the past, errors will continue to be made even with the assistance of computerization and advanced mathematical techniques.** The reason for this is that computer programs and mathematical models such as inferential statistics are human inventions, just as the incorrect conclusions drawn from observations are the products of human perception. And humans, whether working with or without technology, are fallible. It is also difficult to accept the notion that all science is a human invention and, therefore, is never completely "value free."

The Nature of Scientific Revolutions

■GENERAL CONCEPTS

Scientific revolutions are difficult for both scientists and practitioners, even when they occur rather gradually. Experts in a field often are reluctant to hand their authority over to newcomers who have become "experts" in a different way, through a different training path. Instead of carrying on and adding to traditional ways of thinking, these newcomers will cast doubt on old ways of understanding the world as they introduce new scientific paradigms.

For many years, philosophers of science took the position that sciences grow by accretion, i.e., in an incremental or cumulative manner, with each new bit of knowledge adding to what was known or discovered previously. While sciences sometimes grow by accretion, it is now clear that major advances in science occur typically through scientific *revolutions* rather than incremental knowledge.

The term **revolution** suggests a dramatic departure, if not rejection, of earlier beliefs. The nature of scientific revolutions has been described well by Kuhn (1962, 1974). Revolutions are characterized by a complete *shift* in thinking. In physics, a dramatic shift, a scientific revolution, occurred when Einstein challenged Newtonian physics with his theory of relativity (1938). A scientific revolution occurred in astronomy beginning with Copernicus, and followed by Tycho Brahe and Kepler, all of whom postulated that the earth revolved around the sun rather than vice versa (Dobrzycki, 1978). Cohen (1985) presents the argument that a great revolution in science occurred in the nineteenth century with the emergence of statistics and proba-bilistic reasoning.

■HALLMARKS OF SCIENTIFIC REVOLUTIONS

Kuhn (1962) described scientific revolutions as the result of anomalies that cannot be explained adequately by existing the-ories and, thereby, jettison a field of science into a state of cri-sis. Scientists experience crises when their theories fail to hold up to the challenge of new events or observations.

Sometimes new tools must become available before obser-vations can be made that create a crisis. Consider the invention of the microscope (and the many parallels that can be made with present imaging techniques). At first, Leeuwenhoek's in-vention attracted little attention, and little importance was placed on the microscopic creatures he observed. Later, Pas-teur's work on the relation between microorganisms (visualized through the microscope) and disease was revolutionary for both the understanding of infectious diseases and clinical practice. Prior to this work, surgeons scoffed at the notion of a sterile en-vironment in the operating theater. Anecdotes abound about surgeons who undertook operations without washing their hands and who inspected open incisions while smoking cigars and flicking ashes over the operating table (de Kruif, 1996; Lyons & Petrucelli, 1987). Pasteur's work lent credence to Lis-ter's demand for use of antiseptics in the operating theater, a practice that dramatically reduced patient mortality. In this ex-ample, the visualization of microorganisms plus scientific ob-servations of their lethal effects created a crisis in medicine, resulting in revolutionary change in hospital procedures.

Along with new tools come new concepts and new language necessary to express the concepts. In the above example, organ-isms whose existence were not previously known required names when they were discovered through visualization. To carry this example a step further, the use of the compound microscope along with special staining techniques, contributed dramatically to the science of cytology, including the identification of an array of cancer cells, all of which required names. Consistent with the need for new language accompanying the emergence of new technologies, the National Institute of Nursing Research (1993) identified as its first goal the establishment of a nursing language, including classification systems and taxonomies, and standard language for nursing data.

Cohen (1985) suggested four kinds of evidence for the occurrence of a revolution in science:

1. The judgment of scientists who are active at the time the revolution is occurring
2. Adoption of the new ideas, as evidenced in relevant literature such as articles and textbooks
3. The judgment of historians of science and philosophy who focus on recent events as well as the past
4. The general opinion of scientists working in the field at the present time

These four kinds of evidence can provide valuable information on the question of whether new events or observations have shaken the field sufficiently to command the attention of experts and to appear in respected publications.

Try applying these criteria to the informatics revolution in medicine. If new ideas had not inundated the literature, there would be no need for books (like this one) to help make translations. Adoption of new ideas into practice is happening at an amazing rate, including computerization of hospitals and management of intensive care units with real-time data capture. While many disagreements arise regarding the pro's and con's of this revolution, there is virtually no argument among experts that a revolution exists.

Revolutions in Medicine

■LIFE VERSUS PHYSICAL SCIENCES

Scientific revolutions most typically are thought of as those occurring in the "hard" sciences, such as physics. However, revolutions have certainly occurred in the life sciences as well. Most commonly known in this category is the revolution brought about by the work of Darwin (1859), which continues to engender controversy. Some historians and philosophers of science also identify a revolution in the life sciences emanating from the works of Freud (1953–1974).

One of the most dramatic revolutions in medicine occurred when Harvey, in the seventeenth century, used empirical evidence to challenge Galen's mistaken notions of anatomy and circulation, which had dominated medical thinking for 15 centuries. Based on empirical, quantifiable data, Harvey proposed the notion of a single circulatory system in which the heart pumps blood through the body via arteries and veins. Harvey's work is counted as the first true revolution in the life sciences. The works of Pasteur and Lister discussed above count as life science revolutions as well.

■THE INFORMATICS REVOLUTION

This revolution is not limited to its impact on medicine, since it has affected nearly every aspect of life at the end of the twentieth century and the beginning of the twenty-first. The informatics revolution undoubtedly was triggered by the invention of the first machine regarded as a true electronic computer rather than a mechanical calculator. This machine, known as ENIAC, was revealed to the public in 1946 and was developed largely in response to needs that emerged during World War II. This first "thinking machine" was comprised of more than 17,000 highly unreliable vacuum tubes in addition to resistors, capacitors, relays, and 6000 manual switches. It was eighty feet long and eight feet high. It was designed to perform mundane mathematical tasks, i.e., multiplication and addition and to perform them at incredible speed. ENIAC had been designed to calculate firing tables for the war effort—little additional need for it had been foreseen. Consequently, ENIAC was not "programmable" in the sense that we know programming today. In order to set ENIAC to do a particular calculation, some changing of switches and cables was necessary. While considerable time passed before the advent of programmable computers, ENIAC nevertheless marked the start of the computer age.

The vacuum tube computer was followed by the transistor, and the transistor by the microchip (see Figure 1b). Computers became smaller, faster, more reliable, more versatile, and with the advent of the microchip-based microcomputer in the 1970s, incredibly more accessible. At the start of the twenty-first century, computers are performing everything from mundane billing and banking tasks to making artificially intelligent decisions about medical diagnoses.

■THE INFORMATICS REVOLUTION IN MEDICINE

Certainly, medicine has made use of the new computer "tools," but these tools alone are not solely responsible for the continuing revolution in medicine. The crux of the informatics revolution in medicine is that medical knowledge began to exceed what humans could learn from traditional bedside training as well as what we are physiologically capable of integrating and synthesizing without the assistance of complex mathematical and computer-based tools. The emergence of highly efficient computers allows the vast field of medical knowledge to be captured and constantly

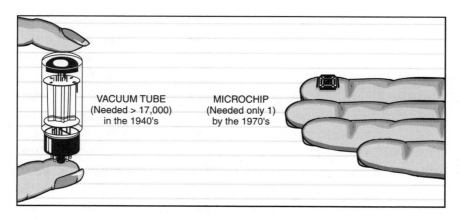

VACUUM TUBE
(Needed > 17,000)
in the 1940's

MICROCHIP
(Needed only 1)
by the 1970's

Figure 1b From vaccum tubes to microchips.

modified and updated. *Medline* permits searching of even the most recent medical literature; *Oncosin* allows physicians to call upon a computerized system to find the leading edge in therapies for their cancer patients; *Illiad* undergoes continued refinement to serve as a second opinion as well as a teaching tool for making medical diagnoses by computer; "real time" data capture permits hospital staff to rely on computers to monitor patient status and to provide immediate warnings when vital signs deteriorate. The World Wide Web permits users to query the National Cancer Institute, the National Centers for Disease Control and Prevention, the Center for National Health Statistics, etc., as well as to obtain via one's desktop computer large health databases from U.S. sources and to "visit" data sites around the globe.

The major problem confronting us is not usually a deficit of information (though on some topics the problem is a deficit of *good* information), but rather the dilemma of how to structure the use and management of all the information that is available. Consider, for example, how easy it is to "lose oneself" while surfing the Web, thereby getting far off track of one's initial purpose in using the Internet. (For more on the Web, see Chapter 7.)

Along with the new tools has come, as anticipated, a new language: supercomputers, mainframes, micros, pc's, laptops, and workstations refer to types of computers; RAM, ROM, cache, hard disks, diskettes, CDs, tape backups, Pentium processors, DVD drives, Zip drives, and MX chip technology are terms that relate to computer memory and computer processing capabilities; Internet, ETHERNET, World Wide Web, twisted pair, modem, FAX modem, and file transfer protocols pertain to information transfer involving more than one machine or "platform"; and communications packages, Windows, operating systems, and word processors are a few examples of types of software, i.e., computer programs. Similarly, the new statistical techniques and mathematical models made possible by high-powered computers continue to introduce their own terms to clinical medicine, i.e., Markov chaining, mutidimensional sensitivity analyses, decision modeling, receiver operating characteristic curves. While this brief sample is by no means a lexicon of informatics terms, it provides a flavor of the language that accompanies the new technologies.

Arguments have been waged against reliance on complex statistical techniques and computers that "learn" and "make decisions." While large sample research, multicenter trials, and meta-analyses may be of great benefit to health care policy, they may provide little guidance for treatment of individual patients. The extent to which summary findings from a large study generalize to an individual patient depends to a great extent on the homogeneity of the sample and the similarity between that individual patient and those who were enrolled in the study. Furthermore, data from most studies do not incorporate measures of patients' values and preferences, so quality of life from the patient's perspective is often omitted. And in a world in which medicine has become increasingly subspecialized and impersonal, patients may fear and resent the loss of human interaction and their physicians' increased involvement in technology. The importance of "bedside manner" tends to slip away as center stage is taken by the seemingly greater importance placed on the physician's ability to enter patients' signs and symptoms properly into the microcomputer on the desk in the consultation office (which probably uploads the information via a networking system to a larger database maintained at the site).

This section on scientific revolutions began with the statement that revolutions are difficult. In medicine, the informatics revolution is difficult for the patient, who often forfeits the more personal interactions associated with medical practice earlier in the past century, and for the health care provider who is required suddenly to become computer literate as well as medically adept.

■THE ROLE OF EVIDENCE-BASED MEDICINE

While both patients and health care providers may struggle with the intrusion of high-tech information systems into their lives, their clinical decision-making abilities can be enhanced by the information that is available through high-tech sources.

Some clinicians believe that the traditional paradigm for acquiring medical skills is in crisis, a crisis that calls into question the reliance on bedside training and amassing experience on a case-by-case basis. The major difference between traditional practice and evidence-based medicine is the new reliance on research literature to inform clinical decisions. This does not mean that health care providers must reject what they have learned from clinical training and experience, but rather that they must also become adept at new skills for accessing and evaluating research literature.

Evidence-based medicine emerged during the 1980s as a system for using medical information to improve everyday health care decisions. The practice of evidence based medicine requires the health care provider to develop a clear statement of the patient's medical problem, search existing medical literature for information pertaining to the patient's problem, evaluate the literature which has been accessed for quality and usefulness, and employ the resulting knowledge to make optimal health care decisions.

Since its introduction, evidence-based medicine has been taught at a number of medical schools, and used to make clinical decisions about individual patients as well as to formulate health care policy for large populations. In 1997 and 1998, the Centers for Disease Control and Prevention (CDC) developed guidelines to evaluate evidence relevant to the prevention and treatment of infection with human immunodeficiency virus (HIV) and the prevention and treatment of tuberculosis (TB) among patients infected with HIV (CDC, 1998a, 1998b; CDC, 1997). The guidelines, which follow principles of evidence-based medicine, are offered below as an example.

Categories Reflecting Strength and Quality of Evidence

In this system, two types of ratings are given. A letter rating signifies the strength of the recommendation. A roman numeral indicates the quality of the evidence supporting the recommendation. This system permits divergent kinds of information about evidence to be captured. For instance, a study might show strong evidence for treatment efficacy, such as a 99% rate of disease prevention. However, the study design might be extremely weak, receiving a poor rating for quality. A combined rating of A, III could be used to rate this evidence.

Letter ratings system for strength of recommendation:
   A.   Both strong evidence for efficacy and substantial clinical benefit support recommendation for use. Should always be offered.
   B.   Moderate evidence for efficacy—or strong evidence for efficacy, but only limited clinical benefit—supports recommendation for use. Should generally be offered.
   C.   Evidence for efficacy is insufficient to support a recommendation for or against use, or evidence for efficacy may not outweigh adverse consequences (e.g., toxicity, drug interactions, or cost of the chemoprophylaxis or alternative approaches). Optional.
   D.   Moderate evidence for lack of efficacy or for adverse outcome supports a recommendation against use. Should generally not be offered.
   E.   Good evidence for lack of efficacy or for adverse outcome supports a recommendation against use. Should never be offered.

Numerical ratings system for quality of evidence supporting the recommendation:
   I. Evidence from at least one properly randomized, controlled trial.
   II. Evidence from at least one well-designed clinical trial without randomization, from cohort or case-controlled analytic studies (preferably more than one center), or from multiple time-series studies or dramatic results from uncontrolled experiments.
   III. Evidence from opinions of respected authorities based on clinical experience, descriptive studies, or reports of expert committees.

Once developed, these guidelines were applied by a committee of experts to the existing modalities for treatment and prevention of HIV, TB, and TB in HIV-seropositive populations. This process resulted in ratings that can be used by clinicians in their daily decisions about treating and preventing TB and HIV disease.

On the down side, evidence-based medicine has been criticized on the point that many clinical decisions have no support from good experimental studies; and that clinicians' judgments and experience must serve, therefore, as the primary arbiter. Weaknesses in evidence-based medicine have been identified in some common adult health problems including acute back pain, hypertension, and screening for vascular disease (Reilly, Hart, & Evans, 1998).

While good evidence might not be available, or even obtainable, for some conditions, good to adequate evidence appears to exist for many medical problems. A retrospective review of 150 clinical decisions contained in charts from a department of internal medicine indicated that most (though not all) therapeutic clinical decisions were supported by randomized controlled trials considered to be good sources of evidence (Michaud, McGowan, van der Jagt, Wells, & Tugwell, 1998). In the same study, for 10 of the 150 clinical decisions considered, the evidence that was found supported other therapies than the ones that had been selected for use. This finding suggests that in a small but clinically significant proportion of cases, evidence-based medicine could have resulted in a better therapeutic decision.

In general, the criticisms that have been made regarding evidence-based medicine have focused on the lack of good evidence available for some, and perhaps many, clinical decisions, rather than inadequacies in the concept itself. These criticisms can be construed as a call for more and better medical information targeting medical therapies that have been under-researched.

Coping with the Revolution in Medical Informatics..............

■ACCEPTING AMBIGUITY AND CHANGE

Since the early 1980s, medical schools and professional organizations have attempted to delineate the domain of study for medical informatics. Models were developed to formalize the numerous and diverse informatics applications, and to define the scope of the field, primarily as a guide to educational programs.

There were different opinions about what the focus of a field of medical informatics should include; different models emerged reflecting these different opinions. Some models focused almost exclusively on the acquisition of computer literacy, while others focused on applications of informatics technology to patient care. To date, no single model of the field has achieved unanimous acceptance.

The report prepared in 1984 by the Panel on the General Professional Education of the Physician and College Preparation for Medicine, appears to have shaped the role of informatics in U.S. medical education more than any other model. The recommendations of that Panel were, generally, to assist students to sharpen and enhance problem-solving skills through the study of medical informatics. The report recommended that for education of all practitioners in the health fields, the following objectives should be incorporated:

- Be able to manage information bases for use in treating patients
- Treat patients more efficiently and cost effectively by using national data bases as references
- Rely on technology to free up physician time to be used on personal aspects of patient care
- Improve the educational process through the incorporation of information technology and decision-making science, as well as computer-assisted instruction

These objectives take on different meanings at the beginning of the twenty-first century than they had in the early 1980s. For example, information technology at that time did not include the massive use of Internet resources for education as well as for patient care. Also, the objectives contain ambiguities, such as how a health care provider should use information bases and national databases to inform treatment.

The field continues to move forward as a collection of techniques and tools that inevitably advance ahead of attempts to generate models that capture clearly what medical informatics is. So, since there is no clear consensus among experts on what constitutes the field, those who are beginning to delve into the ever-changing world of medical informatics must tolerate quite a bit of ambiguity and change. Remember that this elusiveness is a characteristic of medical informatics rather than our personal inability to grasp clearly the scope of the field.

■CONTACTING MAJOR ORGANIZATIONS

One effective route to becoming better acquainted with the field of medical informatics, as well as to keep yourself up to date on its progress, is to attend professional meetings where you can ask questions and see demonstrations of new techniques. Though relatively young, medical informatics has been in existence long enough to spawn a number of organizations dedicated to educational and scientific activities, some of which produce their own publications. While many organizations exist within specialized areas, the focus of this section is to provide information regarding a few general organizations that serve a broad spectrum of health care professionals.

The American Medical Informatics Association (AMIA), based in Washington, D.C., describes itself as the one professional association solely devoted to medical informatics; and it is responsible for the largest U.S. annual meeting in the field. The AMIA meeting is attended by physicians as well as many other health and informatics professionals and provides pre-session workshops and tutorials, as well as scientific paper presentations, demonstrations, and product exhibits. Its international association, the International Medical Informatics Association (IMIA), based in the Netherlands, holds international meetings and sponsors international working groups on special topics. Both AMIA and IMIA produce publications, including newsletters, a yearbook, and a journal. (Note: The AMIA fall meeting has incorporated what once was called the Symposium on Computer Applications in Medical Care, which had been one of the oldest and largest medical informatics organizations.)

The Society for Medical Decision Making, and its *Journal of Medical Decision Making,* began with an almost exclusive focus on decision analysis applications, but has expanded to include other informatics approaches to health care problems. The Society holds an annual meeting at sites across the United States and provides excellent pre-session workshops on informatics techniques. Most sessions and workshops held at meetings of this Society assume a working familiarity with medical informatics and are likely to prove a challenge to beginners. On the other hand, the Society tends to be a showcase for some of the most brilliant informatics approaches to medical questions.

The Society for Judgment and Decision Making, and its *Journal of Behavioral Decision Making,* draws an international audience who target practical applications of decision tools to a range of fields. The scope of this organization is broader than that of the Society for Medical Decision Making; and both presentations and published articles tend to focus less on complex mathematical tools and more on the fit between decision processes and a combination of theory and practice in the social and health sciences. This is a good connection for individuals who are interested in broad informatics applications, without necessarily being interested in catching state-of-the-art advances in formal modeling.

■IDENTIFYING AND PURSUING YOUR OWN GOALS

Understanding medical information during an ongoing revolution in medical informatics can seem an unwieldy and elusive task. Following are some suggestions to assist you in your encounters with medical information and, hopefully, to help make your journey through the field of medical informatics as exciting and enjoyable as possible.

1. When it seems as though you can never quite keep on top of what's happening, remember—you're right! Medical informatics is a thriving, dynamic field, which will make you feel as though you're always playing "catch up." That's the nature of the field, so don't take it personally.

2. Be clear and honest with yourself about what you really need and/or want to know about medical information. While you might need to understand how to translate the results of a Cox regression into a best-guess prognosis for an individual patient, you probably will never need to understand the matrix algebra used by the computer to derive the results.

3. Recognize that state-of-the-art medical information is not about mathematical calculations. Some of the most highly regarded individuals in informatics research would be at a loss if their careers depended on math skills. What is important is to understand the ways in which informatics techniques can provide useable, understandable health care information.

4. When you need help, find books, tutors, and teachers who are compatible with your needs. For example, health care providers and computer programmers typically do not speak the same language, and most computer manuals are unreadable because they have been written by people who spend their time talking to machines. Find teachers and books that address your needs at your level.

5. Learn the language of the new age: Simply knowing what some words mean will enable you to follow a great deal more of what is going on. Learn which terms refer to networking, i.e., linking computers with each other, and which refer to working solo. Separate the terms that refer to a computer's working memory from those that refer to its storage capacity. Familiarize yourself with the

names of the most used software programs for word processing, statistical analysis, and intercomputer communication. And remember that just as there are "name droppers" in the social world, there are "term droppers" in the computer world: The only difference is that in the computer world, people may feign familiarity with chips and networks rather than film stars and political figures.

6. Use the computer market spin-offs to your advantage: Companies are competing to produce user friendly (i.e., intelligible) products and support services. Go for the materials and services that permit you to focus on your task of understanding medical information, instead of forcing you to learn how to program in C++ or how to design software with high-tech graphic capabilities using JAVA.

7. Find newsletters, yearbooks, or journals that help you develop a general sense of what's happening in medical information and what new directions are on the horizon. This will probably be more helpful than reading computer magazines to try to grasp the difference between SX, DX, and MX technology. Consider yourself a consumer of the new technology, and go for a macro-view of the territory—it will most likely prove more valuable than becoming lost in details.

8. Exercise self-discipline when surfing the World Wide Web. The WWW is very seductive; while you got on line with the intention to visit a breast cancer data site in Sweden, you got side tracked along the way by the idea of sending "virtual gifts" to some of your friends. Not good timing if you're serious about getting to that breast cancer data.

9. Exercise self-discipline when surfing the computer stores and catalogues. Remember the old adage *"A sale isn't a sale if you don't need the merchandise."* Like the Web, new technologies can be seductive. If you need more speed and more memory to cope with the data you're presently working with, by all means upgrade! On the other hand, remember that using a new piece of equipment, installing an infrared port or another hard

drive, learning a new software package all take up valuable time. Learn and grow as you need to, and try to adjust your growth to your personal goals and your time availability. Otherwise, you might find yourself spending all your time coping with some new hardware, while that article you thought you would write more quickly on the new machine is nowhere near completion.

10. On the other side of the coin: For readers who do not find the Web or the new technologies seductive, but rather an undesirable drain on time, finances, mental health and brainpower—remember that you will not be able to hold out forever! Try to see the "fun" in the informatics revolution. You might benefit from figuring out why some people have been bitten by the Web and stay up all night surfing it—and then try a little yourself. At the very least, get equipped to use the new communications capabilities. If you decide to keep your usage at a minimum, you will nevertheless welcome the capability to perform vast literature searches from your home computer and to obtain data from files that only a few years ago were accessible only on huge tapes that required mounting on mainframe computers at a university or other large institution.

Summary

Understanding medical information has become more difficult than ever. An unprecedented explosion in medical information has made memorizing and synthesizing information without the assistance of decision tools anachronistic. The information explosion has given rise to sophisticated new tools and techniques for managing and analyzing medical information. Many health care providers believe that there is not enough time in health care curricula to assimilate essential medical information in the field, let alone keep pace with the new technologies. The dilemma, of course, is that a working knowledge of the new technologies is necessary in order to manage the explosion of information.

A brief look at the history of medicine emphasizes the fact that medicine is fallible, and that what is valued as good medicine today may be revealed as bad medicine tomorrow. The history of science shows that the informatics revolution is rather similar to other scientific revolutions. It is characterized by new tools, new language, and changes that have shaken contemporary medicine. It meets the criteria for a scientific revolution, since it already has pervaded textbooks, journals, and curricula. And it has persuaded groups of experts to set new agendas for their particular health fields.

The informatics revolution in medicine affects a broad spectrum of health care providers and is not limited to physician subspecialists or medical informatics professionals. The revolution is difficult for patients as well as for scientists and practitioners: There seems to be less time for "bedside manner" and increasingly more time devoted to data entry. While one goal of contemporary medicine is to involve all health care providers and consumers more actively in health care decisions, difficulties in learning high-technology management and analysis of medical data seem to contraindicate that goal. Furthermore, integrating informatics into health care curricula runs counter to a well-entrenched legacy of reliance on bedside training.

Emphasis on evidence-based medicine requires the health care practitioner to be able to define a patient's medical problem with sufficient accuracy to serve as a sound basis for searching the relevant literature. The health care provider must be skilled in search methods that typically involve using the Internet. Evidence-based medicine also requires the health care provider to be skilled in evaluating the quality of often highly technical research literature in order to decide what constitutes good evidence for medical action.

For health care providers, involvement in professional organizations devoted to scientific and educational activities in medical informatics may prove helpful. To understand medical information in this age of swift and continuous change, it is crucial to have a sense of how much you need to know and where to set your limits. Medical information and the meta-field of medical informatics are not synonymous with mathematics or computer programming. What is most important for most professionals is a conceptual grasp of the kinds of answers you can get from the various informatics techniques that are available, and to be able to understand these answers in real-life, practical terms. With so little time to spare and so much to learn, focus on those methods and materials that help you reach your goals—and set aside those that require you to jump through mathematical or programming hoops before permitting you access to practical knowledge.

Suggested References

■GENERAL REFERENCES FOR USE THROUGHOUT THIS BOOK

- A good medical dictionary. The "gold standard" is Stedman, T.L. (2000). *Stedman's Medical Dictionary* (27th ed.). Baltimore: Lippincott Williams & Wilkins.
- A general but comprehensive medical manual when you need more than a dictionary, but want less than a textbook on general internal medicine. Again, the gold standard is: Merck Sharp & Dohme Research Laboratories. *The Merck Manual of Diagnosis and Therapy.* (This manual is updated approximately every five years, so purchase the newest version available when you are ready to buy.) Rahway, NJ: Merck & Company, Inc.
- A full-scale textbook of general internal medicine. A good choice is Harrison's which is available now on CD ROM, making it enormously convenient, weighing a mere fragment of the hardcopy text. It is also available on line at www.harrisonsonline.com. Harrison's Plus on CD contains links to the journal articles cited in text, and can be updated. The reference is: Braunwald, E.,

Kasper, D. L., Hauser, S. L., et al (Eds). (2001). *Harrison's Plus: Harrison's Principles of Internal Medicine (15th ed.)*. New York: McGraw-Hill.

■SUGGESTED REFERENCES SPECIFIC TO CHAPTER 1

Cohen, J.B. (1985). *Revolution in science.* Cambridge, MA: The Belknap Press of Harvard University Press. This is a comprehensive text that provides extensive discussions on scientific revolutions spanning the seventeenth through the twentieth centuries. In addition to a highly readable history of scientific revolutions, the book also provides a thorough framework for understanding the meaning of scientific revolutions, as well as the concepts of revolution versus revolution in science. It serves well as a primary resource and also provides a wealth of references for following up areas of interest. Reading this book can truly help make up for a lack of course work in philosophy and the history of science.

Kuhn, T.S. (1962). *The structure of scientific revolutions.* Chicago: The University of Chicago Press. There are many excellent texts on the topic of how science proceeds. However, this one was the classic that turned our notions about science upside down. While Kuhn made some revisions in his theories, and other writers responded to his ideas with both criticisms and agreement, this seminal work is the place to begin. It is highly exciting reading, reads sometimes like a novel, and speaks without hedging about the extent to which successful scientists are threatened by *paradigm shifts,* terminology coined by Kuhn and now part of the common vocabulary of scientists.

Fuller, S. (2000). *Thomas Kuhn: A philosophical history for our times.* Chicago: The University of Chicago Press. For anyone truly interested in the works of Kuhn (both the original work noted above, as well as Kuhn's own revisions), this work by Fuller provides a surprisingly different perspective on the impact of Kuhn's writings. Fuller attempts to find ways that science can move beyond what he views as Kuhn's stifling notions of paradigms.

International Medical Informatics Association. *Yearbook of medical informatics.* (Yearly—get the most recent update.) Published jointly by Geneva: International Medical Informatics Association; and New York: F.K. Schattauer Verlagsgesellschaft mbH. This publication covers progress in the basic areas of medical informatics. Areas covered tend to include education and training; clinical management; advances in patient data/bedside information systems; special issues in diagnosis, decision support, and other state-of-the-art developments. It provides a good overview for anyone wanting to develop an understanding of what's happening in medical informatics using a single resource.

Citations In Text

Association of Physician Assistant Programs. (1989). *Physician assistants for the future.* Alexandria, Virginia: Association of Physician Assistant Programs.

Centers for Disease Control. (1997). USPHS/IDSA guidelines for the prevention of opportunistic infections in persons infected with human immunodeficiency virus. *MMWR, 46,* RR-12:1-46.

Centers for Disease Control. (1998a). Report of the NIH panel to define principles of therapy of HIV infection and guidelines for the use of antiretroviral agents in HIV-infected adults and adolescents. *MMWR, 47,* RR-5:1-63.

Centers for Disease Control. (1998b). Prevention and treatment of tuberculosis among patients infected with human immunodeficiency virus: Principles of therapy and revised recommendations. *MMWR, 47,* RR-20:1-53.

Cohen B.J. (As in the preceding Suggested References.)

Darwin, C. (1859). *On the origin of species by means of natural selection, or the preservation of favoured races in the struggle for life.* London: John Murray.

de Kruif, P. (1996). *Microbe hunters.* New York: Harcourt.

Dobrzycki, J. (Ed.). (1978). *On the revolutions.* Baltimore: The Johns Hopkins University Press.

Einstein, A., & Infeld, L. (1938). *The evolution of physics: The growth of ideas from early concepts to relativity and quanta.* New York: Simon & Schuster.

Flexner, A. (1910). *Medical education in the United States and Canada: A report to the Carnegie Foundation for the Advancement of Teaching.* Boston: Updyme.

Freud, S. (1953–1974). *The standard edition of the complete psychological works of Sigmund Freud.* (J. Strachey, Trans). London: The Hogarth Press.

Institute of Medicine. (1995). *Dental education at the crossroads.* Washington, DC: National Academy Press.

International Medical Informatics Association. (1994). *Yearbook of Medical Informatics* Geneva: Internal Informatics Association; and New York: F.K. Schattauer Verlagsgesellschaft mbH.

Kuhn, T. (1962). (As in the preceding Suggested References.)

Kuhn, T. (1974). Second thoughts on paradigms. In F. Suppe (Ed.). *The structure of scientific theories.* Urbana, IL: University of Illinois Press.

Lyons, A. S., & Petrucelli, R. J. (1987). *Medicine: An illustrated history.* New York: Harry N. Abrams, Inc.

Michaud, G., McGowan, J. L., van der Jagt, R., Wells, G., & Tugwell, P. (1998). Are therapeutic decisions supported by evidence from health care research? *Archives of Internal Medicine, 158,* 15, 1665-1668.

National Center for Nursing Research. (1993). Nursing informatics: Enhancing patient care. In the series: *National nursing research agenda, Developing knowledge for practice, Challenges and opportunities.* Bethesda, Maryland: National Center for Nursing Research. (NIH publication number 93-2419).

Panel on the General Professional Education of the Physician and College Preparation for Medicine. (1984). *Physicians for the twenty-first century: The GPEP report.* Washington, DC: Association of American Medical Colleges.

Reilly, B. M., Hart, A., & Evans, A. T. (1998). Evidence-based medicine: A passing fancy or the future of primary care? *Disease-a-Month, 44,* 8: 370-399.

Rootenberg, J.D. (1992). Information technologies in US medical schools. *Journal of the American Medical Association, 268,* 21, 3106-3107.

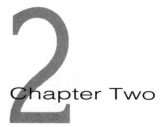

Chapter Two

The Nature of Medical Reasoning and the Limits of Medical Information

Physicians have considerable difficulty collecting and interpreting information from patients, dealing with the uncertainties associated with diagnosing and treating their patients,
communicating precisely with one another, keeping up to
date, and applying recommended procedures when indicated.
Some of the advances in information technology may help
physicians to manage information more effectively. . . .
R. Brian Haynes, Michael Ramsden, K. Ann McKibbon,
Cynthia J. Walker, & Nancy C. Ryan

There is more to heaven and earth, Horatio, than is dreamt
of in your philosophy.

Shakespeare

Introduction

The terms *medical information* and *informatics,* along with associated statistical and computer terminology, seem to suggest that
medical information is **objective**—in other words, clear, unambiguous, quantifiable as well as value-free and unbiased. Before
using the tools and techniques that comprise informatics, it is
critical to recognize that even in this heyday of medical informatics, at the epicenters of high-tech medicine in Western cultures,
there remains a significant component of **uncertainty** in many if
not most medical decisions. In fact, one of the outstanding as-

pects of the revolution in medical information is the emergence of tools and techniques that assist in making medical decisions under conditions of uncertainty. Without uncertainty, the sophisticated informatics tools that have been developed to assist in making diagnoses (e.g., computerized expert diagnostic systems), treatment choices (e.g., decision analysis), and prognoses (e.g., Cox regressions) would be unnecessary.

Medicine has been called an art as well as a science. The term "art"often is invoked when medical decisions cannot be made on the basis of objective information alone, because all necessary information is not available or because factors that are not clearly objective play a significant role in medical choices and outcomes. Why do some patients suffering from a terminal illness seek physician-assisted suicide, while others with the same diagnosis opt for "heroic" medical measures if only to gain a few more months of life? What accounts for the fact that a brilliant diagnostician with a subspecialty in liver disease figured out that a clergyman hospitalized for two decades with a diagnosis of psychosis was in fact a victim of a reversible liver condition that required only a change in diet to achieve normal cognition and release from the hospital after only two weeks?

What often has been labelled art in medicine is an intangible ability of some physicians to arrive at brilliant insights under conditions of great uncertainty in the absence of definitive objective data. To begin to understand the nature of medical reasoning, one needs to come to grips with the fact that the ultimate "instrument" of medical decisions remains the human being. Medicine cannot escape a substantial dose of **subjectivity** because medicine remains a science of some uncertainty, and because medical decisions typically involve values in addition to facts. Each human being who studies, practices, or is a consumer of contemporary medicine is to some extent a product of medical science, as well as a product of his or her culture, individual experiences, ethical and/or religious beliefs, political stance, and a myriad of other factors that make individuals unique.

At least part of what for lack of a more precise term has been labeled the art of medicine is no doubt the sum of the factors mentioned above, brought to bear on medical reasoning. That is, while the physician functions with a body of factual knowledge that is shared at least within a particular subspecialty, each physician also functions with a unique database comprised of a lifetime of experiences, many of which at first glance may not appear to bear a relation to clinical medicine. Furthermore, the physician may be unable to articulate clearly the full thinking process that led to a particular diagnosis or treatment decision, because some things do become "second nature" and are not necessarily accessible on reflection. In other words, a physician, particularly an expert physician, may be unable to access and articulate all the cognitive connections that led to a particular diagnostic or therapeutic insight. Western cultures have chosen to label these intangibles "art." Some other cultures have labeled them "magic." Many cultures view them in a religious context. Daring to paraphrase loosely the Great Bard, there is more to the practice of medicine than is contained in our textbooks or our computers.

There are many categories of decisions made by health care providers. These include decisions about research projects, decisions about policy, and decisions about diagnosing and treating individual patients. The focus of this chapter is the last category: decisions involved in the everyday practice of clinical care.

Medicine as a Science of Uncertainty

■SOLVING MEDICAL MYSTERIES

"I found it only because I was looking for it."
"What? You mean you were expecting to find it?"
"I thought it not unlikely."

Sir Arthur Conan Doyle

Clinical medicine is rarely an exact science, rarely a science in which unambiguous "yes" and "no" answers abound. Instead, it is primarily a science that relies heavily on estimates, in which answers to medical questions most frequently take the form of **probabilities**. It may be highly probable that a young woman's chest pain is due to her chronic bronchitis, but there may be a small yet important probability that the pain has a cardiac cause. Her physician cannot provide an unequivocal "yes" response to the question of whether the chest pain is a product of chronic bronchitis until cardiac causes are ruled out. And even if a cardiac problem is found, it is also possible that the patient's chest pain is caused by both pulmonary and cardiac problems—or by neither, if she perhaps has strained some muscles in what seemed to be a minor fall.

Diagnoses, treatment decisions, and prognoses often involve a substantial degree of uncertainty. A working diagnosis essentially is a hunch played out by a physician with the assistance of medical tests as well as information obtained during the unfolding clinical course of a disease. Frequently, there is a mystery to be solved, but unless the questions are in the realm of forensic medicine, the mystery is not a "who done it" but rather "what's doing it."

Consider, for example, a medical mystery that presented itself during the early 1980s: Young men began to appear in hospital emergency rooms with a collection of nonspecific symptoms, including fever of unknown origin, unexplained weight loss, lymphadenopathy, and varying evidence of suppressed immunity. With this collection of signs and symptoms, but no known disease likely to be responsible, the condition was dubbed Acquired Immunodeficiency Syndrome, i.e., AIDS. Unlike the term *disease,* which implies a known cause, a syndrome typically is a description of a condition, usually a collection of symptoms, with cause unknown. In the unfolding mystery of AIDS, researchers finally identified the human immunodeficiency virus (HIV) as "what's doing it."

During the period between the identification of AIDS and the discovery of HIV, many hunches were followed, some very far removed from the actual cause of the syndrome. These hunches included the hypothesis that inhalation of "poppers," a street form of the drug amyl nitrate, was causing AIDS via the respiratory system. The error in this hunch, of course, was mistaking correlation for cause: Many of the gay men who presented with AIDS used poppers during sex; but HIV turned out to be a sexually transmitted disease (STD), having nothing to do with the street drug commonly used to intensify the sexual "rush."

Breast cancer is a disease, not a syndrome. The cells that comprise the cancer can be viewed definitively on microscopic examination after biopsy or surgery. The existence and proliferation of cancer cells are, in fact, the disease: In such cases, the direct observation of data (cancer cells) establishes the diagnosis of breast cancer. On the other hand, there remains an unsolved mystery behind the solved mystery of diagnosis: What caused the cancer cells to develop and proliferate in the first place? Current investigations suggest that perhaps ten percent of breast cancers are inherited via breast cancer genes. If not genetics, what triggers the development of breast cancer in the remaining ninety percent of cases? Or, are there other "cancer genes" yet to be discovered?

Searching for the cause of a medical problem often has provided the key to successful treatment and sometimes to elimination of the disease. However, the discovery of an effective treatment may lag far behind discovery of the cause. Tuberculosis, which was documented as early as 5000 B.C. (Bartels, 1907), was responsible for one in five deaths in London by the mid-seventeenth century (Ryan, 1993), and claimed the lives of many artists, writers, and composers, including Chopin, Keats, and Chekhov. A number of hunches were followed in attempts to solve the mystery of tuberculosis, earlier known as consumption, including a favored belief that the coughing of arterial blood, fever, weakness, and often death were caused by "bad air" typically found in the dwellings of the poor, among them the struggling creative individuals in cities such as Paris, London, and New York. The discovery of the tubercle bacillus by Koch in 1882 corrected that mistaken belief. Yet, it was the middle of the twentieth century before effective medical therapies to treat tuberculosis began to appear.

■MAKING MEDICAL BREAKTHROUGHS

Chance favors only the prepared mind.

Louis Pasteur

Scientific revolutions, as discussed in Chapter 1, may occur somewhat by chance, as when Pasteur's work on microorganisms and disease reaped the benefits of Leeuwenhoek's invention of the microscope, which made microbes visible for the first time. This, in turn, lent credence to Lister's position that antiseptics were essential in order to prevent infection during surgery. This serendipitous coinciding of medical advances changed drastically the practice of surgery and the rate of surgical mortality through the introduction of sterile precautions in the operating theater.

There continue to be medical breakthroughs that occur under somewhat similar circumstances, involving the play of chance and serendipity. A researcher might not be seeking the cure for a disease, but in the course of investigations done for other purposes might identify something that has broad treatment applications. On the other hand, a scientist or clinician might have a particular goal in mind and pursue that goal successfully in a logical, straightforward manner. In other words, medical reasoning proceeds along diverse paths, and medical advances are made both by accident as well as by carefully planned investigations.

To illustrate some alternate paths in medical reasoning, this section focuses on three classic problems: the need for pain control (i.e., the story of anesthesia), the need for an antibiotic (i.e., the discovery of penicillin), and the control of an infectious disease (i.e., the spread of cholera).

The Story of Anesthesia

In addition to lack of antiseptic procedures, the "other" great problem which confronted early surgeons was the lack of effective pain control. Without pain control during surgery, not only were patients subjected to agony, but also were faced with a high risk of death from pain-induced shock. To get a sense of the human side of this experience, read the description of a mastectomy performed without anesthesia, based on a letter written by the patient in 1811, and incorporated in the historical novel *The Blue Flower* (Fitzgerald, 1997). Particularly chilling is the matter-of-fact discussion of how all neighbors within a certain radius would need to be informed of the impending surgery in order that the screams and cries would not be mistaken for a crime, perhaps a murder.

As early as 1772, nitrous oxide gas was discovered by Joseph Priestley. The gas quickly was dubbed "laughing gas" due to its obvious properties and came into use for social amusement. In other words, nitrous oxide was used as a recreational drug. A contemporary of Priestly, Humphry Davy, noticed that nitrous oxide appeared to have pain-reducing properties. However, his observation regarding nitrous oxide was not taken seriously and failed to prompt an exploration of its use in surgery. In other words, the perception of nitrous oxide as a vehicle for social amusement, as well as the fact that its discovery was not prompted by the search for anesthesia, appears to have put blinders on medical reasoning regarding the use of the gas during surgery.

By 1831, not only nitrous oxide gas, but also ether and chloroform had been discovered. However, scientists who isolated these gases had not been engaged in the search for anesthesia, and did not consider the possible pain-reducing properties of their discoveries.

It is interesting that the push for recognition of the pain-reducing properties of these gases is attributable to two dentists, whose stories are well-worn anecdotes in the history of medicine. The first, Horace Wells, had performed an extraction on himself using nitrous oxide gas, with favorable results. In 1844 he demonstrated the use of nitrous oxide gas for an extraction on one of his patients for an audience of medical students at Harvard. During the procedure, the patient cried out for a reason not clearly known. Assuming that the demonstration of painless extraction had failed, the audience booed Wells, vigorously mocking his concept.

Motivated by a similar goal, Wells' friend and colleague, William T. G. Morton, also a dentist, experimented with the use of ether's pain-reducing properties. In 1846, Morton gave the first public demonstration of surgery without pain using ether. This time, the surgical community took note, and the use of anesthesia complemented the use of antiseptics to enhance greatly the success of surgical procedures.

Why did it take nearly three quarters of a century for the pain-reducing properties of these gases to be recognized and applied as anesthesia? And why was it dentists, rather than physicians, who pioneered and promoted the use of these gases? One speculation is that the job of the dentist was made profoundly difficult in the absence of anesthesia, a practical problem which could very likely have prompted efforts to solve the dilemma. Unlike other body parts, the jaw is extremely difficult to immobilize. It can be virtually impossible to enter the oral cavity without patient cooperation. In addition, candidates for nondental surgeries tended to require such procedures as amputations for fulminant infections, which had rendered them extremely ill and weak. Patients treated by dentists could be quite hearty and able to use their energies to resist dental procedures.

Here, then, is an outline of medical reasoning that progressed by starts and stops, began in laboratories of scientists whose interests lay in domains other than pain reduction, and in a society whose perception of the discovered gases was limited largely to recreation. The problem-solving thread, the thread of medical reasoning, was picked up later by individuals with a specific goal in mind: the application of available drugs (whose pain-reducing qualities had been discovered by accident) to achieve anesthesia.

The Discovery of Penicillin

The events that ushered in the era of antibiotics were remarkable in the extent to which chance played an extremely significant role. Sulfa drugs were the first systemic drugs effectively used to fight bacterial infections in humans. However, since the advent of antibiotics, sulfa drugs have been replaced by these more effective substances.

In 1928, Alexander Fleming discovered something that he believed would be of interest to other researchers engaged in investigations of the nature of bacteria. While working in his lab, Fleming had found that a petrie dish accidentally had become contaminated with an airborne mold, *penicillium*, which inhibited the growth of bacteria in the areas of the mold colonies. As a result of this accidental finding, Fleming went on to explore and demonstrate the efficacy of penicillin, an extract from the *penicillium* mold, to kill many different types of disease causing bacteria in laboratory cultures. He did not extend his work to explorations of the use of penicillin for treating diseases in humans or other animals.

During the winter of 1940–1941, Howard Florey and Ernst Chain widened the door to antibiotic therapy by using penicillin in the treatment of human wounds, including war casualties. This marked the first time that a safe, broad-spectrum agent was available for combating serious infections.

What accounts for the fact that more than a decade elapsed between the isolation of penicillin as an effective antibacterial agent and its use in clinical treatment? First, Fleming, a laboratory bacteriologist rather than a clinician, was "biased" in the applications which he could make of penicillin. Second, the pressing need for effective treatment of infections accompanying injuries sustained during World War I presented an environment in which the search for a clinically useful antibiotic was intensified. Thus, the contexts in which Fleming as well as Florey and Chain worked colored the nature of the advances they made. Said another way, two separate kinds of reasoning processes were responsible for the emergence of penicillin as a therapeutic option: First, Fleming made a chance discovery which, given the "prepared mind" of a brilliant microbiologist, was not ignored but rather appreciated as an inroad into the control of bacteria in the laboratory. Second, Florey and Chain, clinical researchers with a clear goal in mind, responded to the desperate needs of their wartime environment by pioneering the use of penicillin in human medical care.

The Spread of Cholera

John Snow was a British physician whose work on the prevention of cholera stands as a landmark in a branch of medical reasoning known as epidemiology. During the late 1840s, Snow became interested in the problem of cholera, an outbreak of which had occurred in the Soho area of London from which he drew some of his patients. Snow had observed that the outbreak was confined to a small area of the city, an observation which lent credence to his already formulated hypothesis that cholera was spread by contaminated water, since the locale of the outbreak was served by a single water source.

Snow persuaded authorities to remove the handle from the pump which supplied the contaminated water. This action appears to have prevented additional cases and/or a secondary outbreak from the contaminated source. His investigation into the cause of the cholera outbreak actually constituted a test of his hypothesis, which had been formulated through observation of the relation between a well-defined geographic locale and cases of a disease.

Quite unlike the reasoning involved in the examples of anesthesia and penicillin described above, the identification of the cause of cholera owed not to chance but rather to immense creativity, careful observation and, finally, a "test" of an hypothesis to establish its scientific truth.

The Impact of Uncertainty on Medical Information................

> In this world nothing can be said to be certain,
> except death and taxes.
>
> Benjamin Franklin

■OVERVIEW OF THE ISSUES

The complexity of medical problems very often is greater than the capacity of human reasoning to deal with them, even when humans are assisted by the newest informatics tools. Is this because disease processes have become more complex? Probably not. While it is true that some new and very puzzling diseases have been discovered, such as AIDS, Alzheimer's disease, and Ebola Zaire, these discoveries are the exception rather than the rule. Furthermore, it is highly likely that most diseases have been with humankind for ages, but were not identified as specific disease entities. For example, AIDS might have made its way into the path of recognition—and mass contagion—with the opening of the Kinsasha "highway" in Central Africa. Some researchers have speculated that AIDS probably killed off many isolated villages, perhaps over the course of many centuries, but had found no route of transmission beyond these small populations until outsiders began to travel into and out of areas inhabited by the otherwise quiescent virus.

The complexity of today's medical problems, paradoxically, is the result of increased knowledge about diseases as well as increased availability of methods to diagnose and treat disease. With more options for diagnostic testing come more questions about which test is the "best" to perform for a particular patient. With more options for treating disease come more questions about which treatment is optimal for a specific patient, considering both life expectancy and quality of life. Instead of dying very early from mass contagions called plagues, from minor infections such as dental abscesses that could not be treated, from childhood illnesses that are now prevented by inoculation, and from such everyday events as childbirth, humans are living long enough to experience more varied diseases and are expecting medicine to ensure a good quality of life.

The questions of which diagnostic test to select or which treatment to pursue arise from the dilemma that while medical knowledge and technology have reached an all-time highpoint, medicine remains far from perfect. As is discussed in detail later in this book, medicine is full of trade-offs: The tests that are best for diagnostic purposes are frequently the most risky, most uncomfortable, and most expensive. Treatment options that are most effective at arresting or curing a disease often pose the greatest risk to the patient and, again, tend to be the most uncomfortable and expensive. With more diagnostic and treatment choices, there is more room for patients' values and preferences as well as physicians' biases to come into play in medical decisions. (For years now, the *New England Journal of Medicine* has featured regularly a section called "clinical problem-solving" that often deals with an abundance of options. Data about a real patient are presented to an expert clinician in stages; the clinician responds with a reflection on his/her reasoning at each step in the problem-solving process.)

Finally, individual differences among patients account for a great deal of the variation in outcomes achieved through medical intervention. Even when a disease is diagnosed correctly and an optimal therapy is available, a great deal of uncertainty may remain regarding prognosis. A man diagnosed with primary hepatocellular carcinoma (cancer of the liver) may be expected to survive only a matter of months, but may outlive his prognosis by several years. A middle-aged woman diagnosed with advanced (metastisized) colon cancer undergoes surgery and extensive chemotherapy, with a life expectancy of no more than 2 years; 10 years later she is living a full and productive life. Two women diagnosed with Stage II breast cancer at the same age and time follow divergent clinical courses in spite of identical therapies: One woman dies in 24 months while the other shows no residual evidence of disease a decade after diagnosis.

While both clinical and research medicine rely to a great extent on calculations, equations, and mathematical models derived from local as well as national and international databases, and while medical informatics has proven itself to be a health-enhancing field, there persists, nevertheless, a great deal of uncertainty in contemporary medicine. Its presence is obvious in the lack of exactitude and the imprecision in our ability to make prognostic judgments, as well as sure-fire diagnostic conclusions and therapeutic choices. It is expressed in such statistical and informatics terms as standard deviations, probabilities, sensitivity analyses, and error bands. On a more ethnographic level, it is present in the uniqueness of each patient and each physician, just as it is present in the limits of our comprehension of the natural world. Understanding the role of uncertainty in the practice of modern medicine is a critical component in understanding the benefits as well as the limits of state-of-the-art medical information.

■HELP FROM THE PHYSICAL SCIENCES

Perhaps because the practice of medicine has such a personal and immediate impact on individual lives, both patients and physicians are uncomfortable with the somewhat novel and recent revelation that medicine is a science of uncertainty. After all, the application of "informatics" as a way of managing the information explosion in medicine is barely two decades old. In the physical sciences, researchers have been grappling with uncertainty for nearly a hundred years. Concepts of relativity, indeterminancy, and chaos reach back to the first part of the twentieth century (e.g., Einstein, 1938; Heisenberg, 1958) and continue to inform contemporary research. **What do these concepts mean in the physical sciences, and how do they relate to the task of understanding medical information?**

Perhaps these concepts can be summarized as meaning that old notions of cause and effect, and particularly the notion that understanding something leads to an ability to control its outcome, no longer fit many aspects of the universe as we know it. These concepts relate to medical information in the sense that in many areas of medical knowledge, we can speak only in terms of **probabilities,** not in terms of certainties. There are things we cannot predict and/or control because chaos reigns in both the "hard" sciences as well as the life/health sciences: Both have been undergoing similar patterns of change as attention is directed toward increasingly complex problems. This similarity should not be terribly surprising because the physical sciences and the physical person are part of the same universe.

Astronomy and Infections

Astronomy bears interesting parallels to some aspects of medical research, particularly to the branch of epidemiology that uses observation to describe the behavior of diseases, with particular emphasis on infectious diseases and contagion. (See example presented earlier in The Spread of Cholera.)

To begin with, astronomy is one of the "purest" of the hard sciences. It is essentially limited to observation, with no manipulative control over any of the astronomical bodies. In its earliest stages, the movements of the heavenly bodies were understood only poorly, and myths were generated to explain what could not be explained in the absence of appropriate models. Similarly, before infections could be attributed to disease models based on the action of bacteria, they were explained by notions of "bad humours" or "bad air," and treated by rest cures, the application of leeches, bleeding, and other ill-advised methods.

The advent of mechanical models in astronomy brought major change in that they effectively predicted action at a distance—the movement of planets in our solar system. The microbe model of infection worked well to explain some disease processes in medicine, and it brought about the recognition that what could not be seen previously with the naked eye was nevertheless the cause of morbidity and mortality. What is interesting about these parallels is that both astronomy and the study of infection have struggled with extremes of measurement: Astronomy deals with immense bodies at unimaginable distances; research on infection deals with entities so small that they are visible only with the aid of strong magnification. The two areas of study essentially look through the opposite ends of the optical glass, both requiring great visual power.

Mechanical models also assisted medical progress because they provided ways in which such essential processes as the circulation of blood could be understood. However, in medicine as in astronomy, what was being achieved were new models for understanding or describing their subjects, not models for intervention or control. And while these new models were far better than the old ones for some kinds of prediction, they were not perfect or devoid of uncertainty. In fact, as the complexity of the subjects under study became more apparent, the initial models failed.

So, mechanical models of the solar system worked quite well, particularly after hitches regarding the elliptical orbits of planets were worked out using somewhat more refined mathematical models. The great challenge to the mechanical models of astronomy came when improved telescopes showed the existence of galaxies other than our own and alluded to problems of measurement on an even grander scale, far too large and complex for existing models. When physicists began to study these complex problems in astronomy, they found that a notion of a mechanical universe where everything is fixed and known with certainty, and that can be calculated exactly, no longer worked. Thus, physics moved into the relativistic era in which mass, energy, and time are viewed as interrelated and variable depending on the conditions under which they exist.

Issues of relativity came into the foreground with the study of light, under the rubric of quantum theory. Light, which had been thought of as a wavelength, was seen also to have properties of solid matter (photons, gamma rays) depending on varying circumstances. The speed of light appeared to be its only constant. Scientists Einstein and Bohrs developed and used a new mathematics to generate relativistic models of the universe that could better explain such things as the behavior of light. The "fixed and known" mechanical model of the universe had broken down when the need arose to explain very complex, relativistic phenomena.

One of the crucial points that contemporary medicine can glean from relativity in physics is that complex systems are characterized by very complex interrelations, which make them difficult if not impossible to predict and control. The physical body, like the physical universe, is extremely complex. While we have begun to find treatments that effectively kill cancer cells, we have been forced to realize that these actions do not occur independent of the rest of the physical system. In fact, many effective "cancer" treatments also kill noncancerous cells necessary to support life. As we have begun to pick up the genetic code of some cancers, we are uncertain as to what effects tampering with the implicated sites on the genome will have for the far-flung health of the individual, not to mention possible unanticipated genetic mutations in the population. If we treat one infection with antibiotics, we may destroy the normal flora of the body, and in the process cause other problems such as vaginal yeast infections. We may also create drug resistant strains of bacteria, as in multiple drug-resistant tuberculosis, which can be highly lethal because they are not sensitive to existing medical regimens.

Thus, the complexity and interrelatedness, which characterize the human body as well as the health of populations, bear much resemblance to the problems of uncertainty and relativity in the so-called hard sciences. If an inability to predict with certainty remains elusive in these other areas, is it surprising to find that the universe of the human body continues to defy errorless prediction?

Out of the Lab, Out of Control

One of the most recent approaches to dealing with the complexity of the world around us is called **chaos theory.** This theory suggests that the factors that impact on any outcome are so complex, that it is impossible to know what the endpoint will be. The classic illustration of this point is the notion that a butterfly flapping its wings in South America can "cause" a change in the weather in New York.

Consider the ways in which chaos might impact in clinical medicine. A physician prescribes a simple diuretic for a 50-year-old woman with mild hypertension. The therapy is known to be effective and benign when taken as prescribed and appropriately monitored by the physician. In other words, under **controlled conditions,** the therapy will work and will do no harm.

One month later, the woman is dead as a result of trauma, indirectly related to her simple, benign diuretic. What went wrong? Chaos—that is, the impact of many factors that could not possibly have been predicted by the woman's physician. First, the patient experienced a slight but persistent dizziness as a result of the diuretic. She was not assertive by nature, and she simply continued to comply with the therapy without discussing this side effect with her physician. A heat wave occurred, which adversely affected the patient who habitually had a low fluid intake and failed to replenish the fluids lost in perspiration. This perspiration fluid loss exacerbated the side effects of her diuretic. In an effort to cool off, she opened the windows and doors to her home. Her house cat ran outside, became frightened by unfamiliar sights and sounds, and climbed a tree. The patient panicked, rose too rapidly from a sitting position, ran to fetch a ladder to rescue her cat, scaled the ladder, became seriously dizzy and fell, sustaining a broken neck. While this example is contrived, it is also quite plausible. At any point in the string of events, other "chaos" phenomena could impinge and alter the outcome: a neighbor passing by catches the cat before it climbs the tree, the patient faints from the effort of carrying the ladder and never uses it, or she gets distracted from her pursuit by someone or something else.

Why are prognoses so difficult to make and filled with error and uncertainty? Prognostic information is based on averages. For example, the "average" person with mild hypertension responds well to a once-daily diuretic. On the other hand, there are many deviations from that "average," deviations relegated to the category of error. What causes error/deviation from the average in clinical medicine? There are many factors, including but not limited to, an individual's unique physiology. Other factors might include personality, life style, and chance events in the environment. Even simple laboratory tests have a built-in tolerance for error. For example, all blood chemistries acknowledge a range of what is considered normal—and this range differs across geographic sites.

The recognition that many factors impinge on medical outcomes has prompted the development of complex models that attempt to make sense of what appears to be chaos. One such approach is pattern recognition, a computerized form of artificial intelligence. Such models have shown some success in reducing the "error" in medical predictions, but have not succeeded in eliminating it.

■THE IMPACT OF BIAS

Medical decisions may be divided into two categories: those which are very clearly life-and-death decisions, as when a patient is brought into an emergency room exsanguinating from a gunshot wound that has nicked an artery; and those which depend to a great degree on quality-of-life issues, such as whether to perform surgery for benign prostatic hypertrophy knowing that the intervention might cause impotence and incontinence (Jordan, et al., 1994).

There tends to be more room for bias on the part of health care providers when the outcomes of treatment involve quality of life rather than life or death. Bias occurs when diagnostic or treatment decisions are made on the basis of factors that are irrelevant to the medical decision. Deciding that an elderly patient with heart disease should not undergo orthopedic surgery on his hand because he faces an unacceptably high risk of heart attack is a decision made on the basis of **health status.** Deciding that an elderly patient does not require orthopedic surgery to repair his hand simply because he is elderly is an instance of **bias.**

Bias in health care decisions may relate to the patient's age, gender, race, and socioeconomic status. Other, less obvious biases, may center on the patient's physical appearance or the etiology of the disease. Some research suggests that health-care providers tend to dislike working with elderly patients. Consequently, decisions made for older patients may be stereotypic, focusing on presenting symptoms and ignoring quality of life in such areas as sexuality (Jordan, et al.,1994). A woman's age and physical attractiveness may impact a physician's recommendation to perform preventive bilateral mastectomy in an effort to avoid breast cancer (Jordan, et al., 1995). Is a patient who has contracted HIV through a blood transfusion treated with the same consideration as one who has contracted the infection through prostitution or through intravenous drug use? Data have shown an unexpectedly high risk of death from preventive therapy for tuberculosis in black women (Jordan et al., 1991). Why, then, did many decision models examining the pro's and con's of preventive therapy fail to investigate the impact on black women specifically?

In the following chapter, an example is provided of the overuse of tonsillectomy, which occurred because pediatricians expected that 50% of all youngsters would need this surgery. This is a classic example of unconscious bias: Pediatricians were not overusing tonsillectomy because they were attempting to harm children, but rather because they were experiencing the impact of a bias that was prevalent among their peers.

Bias distorts judgment, rendering it less than objective. There are three general levels of bias to which humans are vulnerable:

1. *General cultural bias.* This bias refers to beliefs held by the majority culture in which an individual lives. An example of a current bias in the general U.S. culture is that being slim is important.
2. *Group/peer bias.* These are perspectives taken by subgroups with which an individual identifies. Such groups may be socioeconomic, ethnic, occupational, etc. An example of a peer bias is physicians' preference to do something rather than nothing, even if treating a patient holds little hope of cure and entails miserable side effects.
3. *Individual bias.* This refers to a person's idiosyncratic way of looking at the world. An example of an individual bias is a person's adamant belief that general anesthesia is unnatural and should be avoided regardless of the consequences.

There are two great difficulties with bias: First, people typically are unaware of their biases. This is true particularly when the bias is held by their peers or by the general culture. For example, health care providers' jobs are to diagnose, prevent, and treat disease. Consequently, doing something (rather than nothing) is what they expect from each other—even if a patient is highly unlikely to benefit from yet another round of chemotherapy or another try at a liver transplant. Second, many biases have a "grain of truth" in them, which can make them difficult to refute. For example, the cultural bias toward slimness can be "defended" on the basis that being overweight can have negative health consequences. What is missing from this defense is that being underweight can have even greater health consequences.

There are three factors that should be considered when trying to become more aware of the biases which might be distorting our beliefs:

1. *We see what we expect to see.* This is why the pediatricians in Bakewin's study made so many inappropriate decisions for tonsillectomy. They expected children to need the surgery.
2. *We see what others around us see.* This is why we view weight loss positively and weight gain negatively. If we were living in a culture of extreme poverty, in which our children were dying from kwashiorkor, we might see weight gain as a good sign of health and affluence and weight loss as a sign of impending doom.
3. *We see only as much as our physiological apparatus allows us to see.* This is why we need informatics tools, including statistics and decision models. We cannot cope cognitively with hundreds or thousands of pieces of information at a time. Consequently, we need tools and techniques that can assist us in dealing with the information explosion. If we were able to store and manipulate more information "in our heads," we would not need personal computers, personal digital assistants, or even calculators.

■ HINTS FOR DEALING WITH UNCERTAINTY IN MEDICINE

Clearly, health care providers often are uncomfortable with the uncertainty that continues to pervade medical reasoning. Discomfort is compounded when professional colleagues and patients refuse to accept the uncertainty inherent in contemporary medicine and insist on absolute answers. Accepting the unavoidable uncertainties in medical information is essential in order to obtain the best information possible from health care providers, as well as from reports of medical research. Following are some hints for getting the most accurate information from a highly uncertain science:

1. Don't *insist* on "yes" or "no" answers. Absolute answers to medical questions are obtainable only some of the time. Much of the time, both diagnostic and treatment decisions contain elements of uncertainty. If you insist on getting a "yes" or "no" answer to a question that can only be answered accurately with a "maybe," you will wind up getting a distorted picture of what's happening.

2. Develop a healthy suspicion of answers that appear to be perfect, because perfection is extremely rare. Research that reports favorable responses in 100% of the cases, physicians who guarantee that a treatment will work for you or your client, anything that looks "too good to be true" should be regarded with some skepticism and double-checked with other research or authorities in the field.

3. When speaking with a health care provider about a medical decision, don't assume you both hold the same values, biases, or perspectives. Make your values as explicit as possible and ask questions about the criteria the health care provider is using to arrive at his or her recommendation.

Summary

In general, humans are uncomfortable with uncertainty, particularly when the uncertainty has immediate, personal implications. Consequently, it is not surprising that uncertainty in medicine is particularly disconcerting.

It is easy to believe that the information explosion in medicine has heralded a new era in which uncertainty is eliminated by technological advances and sophisticated models for making diagnoses, providing optimal treatments, and generating accurate prognoses. This is not quite the case. In fact, the emergence of more choices in diagnostic testing as well as in treatment options has actually increased uncertainty in many areas of medicine. The sophisticated models, usually quantitative and computer-based, which have been developed under the rubric of "informatics" have actually been attempts to cope with unwieldy amounts of information, great complexity, and great uncertainty in contemporary medicine.

It may seem paradoxical that as medicine progresses, and the body of medical knowledge grows by leaps and bounds, the degree of uncertainty about medical choices increases as well. Does this mean that medical information is poor or useless? Certainly not. Looking to examples in the "hard" sciences, it is clear that recognition of increased complexity, interrelatedness, and chaos is a mark of a maturing science. The medical advances that have brought about greater uncertainty are those that have brought forward new diagnostic modalities and treatment options. The models that cannot provide perfect predictions of medical outcomes are imperfect because there is room for greater variation than ever before in the ways humans respond to medical interventions—people no longer die at very young ages due to relatively simple medical problems, but rather survive to increasingly old ages, experience a variety of now treatable medical problems, and play a more active role in their medical choices.

If, in spite of the above arguments, the limits of medical information still inspire feelings of uneasiness, consider how Einstein felt about physics. He said that, "God does not play dice with the Universe." In this statement, Einstein disclosed his discomfort with a probabilistic universe.

Suggested References

Hahn, R.A., & Atwood, D.G. (Eds.). (1985). *Physicians of western medicine: Anthropological approaches to theory and practice.* Boston: Reidel Publishing Company. This book provides an interesting foray into differing perspectives on contemporary medicine. It includes such chapters as, "How surgeons make decisions" and "Menopause as syndrome or life transition." The book is likely to be of interest to readers who would like to broaden their perspectives of what constitutes health, healing, and illness as seen from the vantage points of different medical subspecialties as well as different cultures.

Katz, J. (1984). *The silent world of doctor and patient.* New York: The Free Press. Physician-patient relationships are the major focus of this book. A great deal of discussion centers on patients' rights and physicians' obligations to communicate effectively. The section on uncertainty in medicine is excellent. The book also provides a good deal of factual information about the history of patients' legal rights, and includes both the 1847 Code of Ethics of the American Medical Association and the 1980 American Medical Association Principles of Medical Ethics.

Riegelman, R.K. (1991). *Minimizing medical mistakes.* Boston, Massachusetts. Little, Brown and Company. This is a book written by a physician for physicians. It gives an "insider's" view of the problems confronting today's physicians, including how to handle uncertainty, how to deal with difficult patients, and how to avoid excessive medical testing. While most of the book is devoted to teaching the process of making correct diagnoses, it ends with a revealing chapter titled, "Facing fallibility."

Schwartz, S., & Griffin, T. (1986). *Medical thinking: The psychology of medical judgment and decision making.* New York: Springer-Verlag. The focus of this book is on the process by which physicians arrive at medical decisions. It provides extensive coverage of relevant theories of cognition and information processing, provides examples of how risks and benefits are evaluated, and ends with a section on formal decision modeling. It is probably the most comprehensive text on the topic of medical thinking.

Citations in Text

Bartels, P. (1907). Tuberculose (Wirbelkaries) in der jungeren Steinzeit. *Archives of Anthropology, 6,* 243-255.

Einstein, A., & Infeld., L. (1938). *The evolution of physics: The growth of ideas from early concepts to relativity and quanta.* New York: Simon & Schuster.

Fitzgerald, P. (1997). *The blue flower.* New York: Houghton Mifflin Company.

Heisenberg, W. (1958). *Physics and philosophy: The revolution in modern science.* New York: Harper & Brothers.

Jordan, T. J., Lewit, E. M., & Reichman, L. B. (1991). Isoniazid preventive therapy for tuberculosis: A decision analysis considering race and gender. *American Review of Respiratory Disease, 144,* 1357-1360.

Jordan, T. J., Grallo, R., & Montgomery, R. (1994). Combining decision analysis and experimental data: The example of benign prostatic hypertrophy. *Journal of Research in Education, 4(1),* 58-67.

Jordan, T. J., Montgomery, R., & De Jager, R. L. (1995). Decision models for treatment of lobular carcinoma in situ. *The European Journal of Cancer, 31a,* Supplement 5:665.

Ryan, F. (1993). *The forgotten plague: How the battle against tuberculosis was won—and lost.* Boston: Little, Brown and Company.

3

Chapter Three

The Realms Of Medical Research

> . . . very little of medicine has been carefully evaluated in well designed, well controlled studies . . . What that means for the patient—and not just for the patient but for the physician—is that for a large proportion of practices we really don't know what the outcomes or what the effects are.
>
> D. M. Eddy

Introduction

The quotation that leads into this chapter is likely to surprise some readers of medical literature. Perhaps the most helpful way to understand Eddy's statement is to understand that medical research is both marvelous and limited. It is true that many crucial advances in medicine have occurred "by accident," or through anecdotal observations of a single case. On the other hand, many medical procedures that are presently thought of as cutting-edge have not been studied under rigorous, scientific conditions. Without such rigor, it is impossible to be certain which treatments yield the best outcomes for which patients, and which diagnostic procedures are best for which diseases. And without this kind of information, the practice of evidence-based medicine has no foundation.

High speed computers, the burgeoning field of medical informatics, high-tech diagnostic and therapeutic machines—these accouterments of Western medicine at the start of the twenty-first century can easily convince us that we should be able to find the "magic bullets" (Konner, 1993) to cure disease. With many advantages at the disposal of contemporary medical

researchers, the consumer of research is left with some disturbing questions: **Why don't we have more or better answers to
our questions about what causes and what cures diseases
such as HIV/AIDS and cancer? And, what prevents medical
research from being as rigorously scientific as we would like it
to be?** There are many answers to these questions, several of
which are discussed below.

■THE PROS—AND CONS—OF ETHICS

In dramatic contrast to research performed only a few decades
ago, medical research today is monitored in an increasingly
careful manner. In order to perform a study in a hospital, university, or other health-care environment, the institution's **Internal Review Board** (IRB) must carefully evaluate the potential
benefits of the research as well as any possible harm it might
cause. Where more than one institution is involved, as in what
is called a "multicenter" trial, IRBs at each institution must approve the research. It is the responsibility of the investigators to
provide detailed information to the relevant IRBs, and to obtain
full approval before embarking on the research program.

The history of IRBs can be summed up by saying that, for
many years, the rights of people (as well as other animals)
often were treated as secondary to research pursuits. In ethical
terminology, much research was pursued from the perspective
that the end justifies the means. In other words, what we learn
will be so valuable that it is worth whatever it takes to get there.
In clinical medicine specifically, there is a long-standing tradition that views the patient's hospital bed as a field of scientific
investigation where the patient is observed much as a laboratory experiment (Foucault, 1994).

It is interesting that one of the strongest pushes for the development of boards to oversee research came from the social
sciences, from Stanley Millgram's work on the authoritarian
personality. Following the atrocities committed during World
War II, Millgram became interested in the extent to which humans can be persuaded to perform unethical and even harmful

acts at the bidding of an authority figure. In brief, his research required human subjects to administer electric shocks to students in a so-called learning experiment. Deception was used in the research: The "students" were research collaborators (called *confederates*) who in actuality were not hooked up to the electric shock machines, but who pretended to suffer pain when subjects worked a mechanism which they were told administered electric shocks. Results revealed that more than 50% of the participants administered extremely high voltage shocks at the request of a senior investigator, even when they heard cries of pain emitted by the "students." Research participants were debriefed after their participation, i.e., they were told that the shocks were fake and that no injury had been caused. However, injury had been caused to the participants: The majority had learned something disturbing about themselves, that they were capable of injuring others simply at the encouragement of an authority figure. Follow-up studies of participants revealed a substantial amount of psychological damage years after the investigation. **This work clearly indicated that debriefing is not enough—and that deception in research can be harmful.**

In the domain of medical research, one of the most infamous breaches of patients' rights can be seen in what is known as the "Tuskegee syphilis study" (See Corbie-Smith, 1999; Jones, 1981). This investigation was designed to track the effects of untreated syphilis on human subjects, with particular attention to the question of whether the clinical course of the disease was different in African American men than in other ethnic groups. A longitudinal study was begun in the 1940s and terminated in the mid-1970s. African Americans enrolled in the study were provided free medical examinations, food, and transportation, as well as burial stipends to families who agreed to autopsies on deceased study participants. This study is the longest (1932–1972) nontherapeutic experiment on humans in the history of medicine.

The critical aspect of this study was that participants who were diagnosed with syphilis during their medical exams were not informed of this diagnosis and were not treated for the

**disease in spite of the fact that it was well known that un-
treated syphilis progresses to neurosyphilis and death.** During
World War II, some of the study participants who were in the
Armed Forces were ordered by the draft boards to undergo
treatment for syphilis; the Public Health Service intervened to
convince draft boards to exclude these men from treatment.
Through the 1970s, the Public Health Service worked with
health departments throughout the South to *prevent* study participants from receiving treatment for their disease.

The nature of the study was brought to public attention in
1972 via the Associated Press and was terminated. When John
Heller, the director of the Venereal Diseases unit of the Public
Health Service from 1943 to 1948 was questioned about the
ethics of the "experiment," he responded that: "The men's status did not warrant ethical debate. They were subjects, not patients; clinical material, not sick people" (Jones, 1981, p. 179).

From studies such as the above, issues of **empowerment**
and of the rights of patients and research subjects came sharply
into focus. To help safeguard the rights of research participants,
investigators now are required to avoid deception and to provide elaborate information about their research. As part of most
research protocols, patients must be given an **informed consent** form to be read and either signed or refused. While informed consent forms differ from study to study, there are
several factors that are required by nearly all IRBs:

1. The language describing the research study must be understandable to the patient who is responding. This
   means that great attention must be paid to the reading
   level as well as the native language of the patient. For all
   patients, the language must be in lay terms, without reliance on medical jargon.
2. The research options must be stated explicitly. This
   means that the form must indicate what will happen if
   the patient opts to participate in the research versus
   what will happen if the patient refuses to participate. The
   patient must be assured that under no circumstances

will treatment be denied if he/she refuses to participate in a study. This may be particularly important for patients who do not carry insurance, and feel "at the mercy" of those who are running the research.

3. Patients must be informed that they have the right to discontinue participation in the study at any point.
4. If the study involves "blinding" (meaning that patients will not be told whether they are in one group versus another, e.g., a treatment versus a control group), this must be made abundantly clear.
5. A primary contact individual must be provided in the event that patients wish to ask questions, discuss side effects, consider other options, etc.
6. Finally, to the best of the investigator's ability, all potential risks to the patients must be spelled out explicitly.

The informed consent essentially is a contract that is designed to give patients right of refusal, as well as full disclosure of the research protocol.

What problems can well-intentioned informed consent procedures cause? One of the most difficult tasks for many medical researchers is to develop a form that meets all the above mandates without sounding unduly negative and scaring away patients who could benefit from the study. Consider the fact that nearly any medication, inoculation or procedure, even the most benign, can cause serious or even fatal effects in rare instances. Benign procedures are very unlikely to cause harm—but unlikely is not the same as never. Therefore, most forms contain a substantial list of undesired effects, from minor discomforts to serious illness and death. Because forms which exhaustively disclose all possible outcomes conscientiously include negative consequences, many possible participants are scared away. Those who elect to participate in the investigation may represent a skewed sample of the population. For example, those who participate may be patients for whom other therapies have not worked; and so they are more willing to take risks in order to get well. What is the impact of such "elective" participation on the study results? If only those patients who have been refractory to existing therapies enlist to participate in the study, they will probably be less likely than others to do well with the new therapy. After all, they have a history of therapeutic failures, a history which may repeat itself. Consequently, the study might end up showing that a new therapy is of no use at all—when very different conclusions might have been drawn from a different sample of patients. Results of the study may discourage further research, thus terminating inquiry into a mode of treatment that could be of great benefit to other patients.

In addition to the role of the IRB at the investigator's home institution, research that is funded by federal agencies, as well as by some private sources, is monitored for ethical problems. One rule that has come to guide medical research is that keeping patients in separate treatment groups is ethical *only* when there is absolutely no indication that any group is doing better than any other group. What does this mean in practical terms? Essentially, it mandates that researchers keep track of patients' progress in an ongoing manner and, if they should see that one group is doing better than others, the research protocol must be halted and all patients must be "crossed over" to the more successful group.

An instance of the above occurred in the American aspirin study, which enrolled middle-aged physicians into a study designed to determine whether taking an aspirin a day would reduce the risk of heart attack (Steering Committee of the Physicians Health Study Research Group, 1989). Participants in the study did not know whether they were enrolled in the treatment (aspirin) group, or whether they were getting a placebo in place of treatment. Partway through the study, the aspirin experiment was terminated because preliminary results suggested that risk of having a heart attack was substantially lower in the aspirin group. At that point, the funding agency halted the study, and all patients were informed of their status as "treatment" or "placebo" so that everyone could benefit from the effects of once-a-day preventive therapy with aspirin.

The early end to this study drew a great deal of attention, particularly because it suggested that aspirin was enormously successful in fighting heart attacks. However, the premature termination of the study can also be criticized on a number of points: First, while the aspirin group showed fewer heart attacks, there was no difference in numbers of deaths due to heart attack in the aspirin group compared with the placebo group. Second, the aspirin group had a higher incidence of serious and/or fatal strokes. Finally, some patients on daily aspirin might eventually develop gastrointestinal disturbances, even on a low aspirin dosage. Terminating the study early stopped the investigators from obtaining further data that might have raised some objections to aspirin. As it stands, consumers of research did not have the benefit of further data from this study. (In the years since the study was terminated, other sources have confirmed the efficacy of aspirin in preventing heart attacks, thereby confirming the early conclusion that "aspirin therapy works.")

■THE ROLE OF HUMAN BIAS IN RESEARCH DESIGN

Thomas Chalmers who had been Dean of the Columbia University Medical School, stated that in his opinion, the greatest advance in medical research in the twentieth century was the development of **clinical trial methodology.** Until rather late in this century, it commonly was believed that there was no need for experimental procedures in clinical research in order to ensure objective, scientific results. Physician researchers were not "blinded" to the treatments their patients received during clinical research; and they performed research evaluations of a patient's progress with full knowledge of his/her medical regimen. This practice had remained unquestioned for many years because physicians were viewed as invulnerable to bias.

In pointing out the importance of changing this view, Chalmers was not accusing his fellow physicians of deliberate unscientific behavior, but rather alerting the medical establishment to the fact that physicians, like other humans, can be unconsciously biased in favor of some results and against others.

For centuries, physicians of Western medicine enjoyed a societal role not unlike priests and priestesses. Suggesting that the opinions of expert physicians, authorities in their fields, could be less than the final word on topics of medical treatment was undoubtedly shocking. However, numerous cases were uncovered that began to lend credence to the notion that new research designs were needed in order to improve medical practice.

An early example of the role of documented bias in physician judgment centered on the widespread practice of performing tonsillectomies on young children. During the 1940s, a New York pediatrician named Bakewin (1945) observed that many youngsters were being subjected to tonsillectomies. The literature at the time suggested that approximately 50% of all children had tonsillitis and, therefore, required this procedure. However, Bakewin suspected that because physicians expected that half of all children needed tonsillectomies, their medical judgments would be biased by what they expected to see.

To study this bias, Bakewin and his colleagues (1945) selected 1000 asymptomatic children from the New York City public schools. He sent these youngsters to a panel of pediatricians, who diagnosed tonsillitis and recommended more than half of the youngsters (661) for tonsillectomy. The remaining children were sent to a second panel of pediatricians. Of this group of 339 children, half again, were recommended for tonsillectomy. The process was repeated two more times, as illustrated in Figure 3a. By the time Bakewin ran out of pediatricians for his exam panels, 985 children of the original 1000 had been recommended for tonsillectomies. Only 15 children had "escaped" this recommendation. (And one can imagine how this number would have been halved yet again and again if more pediatricians had been available.)

What accounts for these findings? In spite of the fact that all youngsters in the study were asymptomatic for tonsillitis, each panel of pediatricians continued to recommend surgery for just about half of the remaining youngsters referred to them. Results of this classic investigation were taken to indicate that physicians, like most humans, see what they expect to see. And since the medical literature fostered a belief that half of all youngsters

Perception and Preconception

The Theoretical Survival of Tonsils after Medical Examination
(Bakwin, 1945)

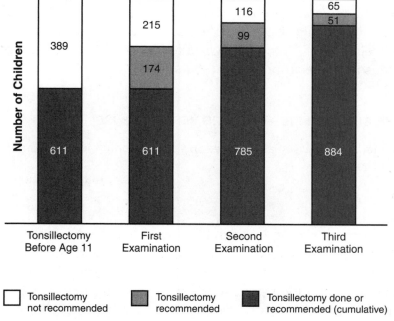

Figure 3a Bakewin's results.

needed tonsillectomies, pediatricians truly believed they "saw" a
need for the procedure in half the children they examined.

The research designs discussed in detail later in this chapter are, in large part, the product of a growing awareness that
the design of studies should build in as many safeguards
against bias as possible. The tonsillectomy example shows a
bias toward seeing something rather than nothing. This bias toward finding meaningful results that are consistent with what is
known or expected can pose major problems not only in clinical practice but also in interpreting results of medical research.

In contemporary medical practice, missing a diagnosis is
identified by the legal profession as negligence, a kind of error

which results frequently in malpractice claims. To avoid negligence, as well as to meet a patient's needs, health care providers look long and hard to find the source of a patient's complaint, since encapsulating the complaint in a diagnosis provides a certain sense of security and direction. Unfortunately, when this pressure is felt too intensely, it can increase the likelihood of "false positive" errors—seeing something when there is no medical problem to be seen.

■THE BOTTOM LINE—DOLLARS VERSUS SENSE

> Medicine is a social science, and politics only medicine on a grand scale.
>
> Rudolf Virchow

Excellent medical research is expensive. Even without considering the costs associated with specific medical therapies, the person-power required to evaluate large groups of patients over sufficiently long periods of time can bear price tags in millions of dollars. Most medical research requires special funding, i.e., funding beyond that which is provided by patients' medical insurance or an institution's regular budgetary allowances. Consequently, the vast majority of medical investigations are funded by sources outside the researcher's home institution. These outside sources most commonly include drug companies, federal agencies, and private foundations.

Since investigators are expected to acknowledge sources of financial support for their work, published articles bear a note (usually in small print on the first page) which informs the reader of any "outside funding" for the research that is being reported. As a consumer of medical research, it is helpful to know who has funded a study because the source of funding can impact on what is—and is not—reported.

Research funded by pharmaceutical companies is performed because drug companies are businesses that need clinical evaluations of their products to be used to market medications. Good research results are good for advertising and good for sales. Reprints of studies reporting favorable results are handed out by drug company representatives at medical conferences to convince physicians to use their products. No one hands out studies reporting unfavorable results. Unimpressive or negative results work against a company's economic interests. This is not to suggest that drug companies fund shoddy or misleading studies. In fact, strong studies yielding favorable results are more desirable than poorly designed ones. However, consider the following caveat: When investigators contract with a drug company to perform research funded by that company, they typically are required to sign a form which gives the company the right to approve or refuse publication of the results. What this often means is that studies which support a company's interests get published, while negative studies are not submitted for publication. If a product performs badly, it will most likely be discontinued quietly in order to avoid poor customer relations. Consequently, the consumer sees one side of the coin: We are permitted to see evidence that a product has worked, but we are not permitted to see dismal failures. Research that is directed too strongly by the pressures of funding from pharmaceutical companies has been criticized also for choosing inappropriate comparisons that inevitably favor their own drugs. **The major lesson here is that it is difficult to get an objective picture of a medication or procedure when the studies you are reading are funded by an economically "interested" party.**

When research is funded by federal agencies, investigators typically are required to sign a very different kind of form—a disclosure of **conflict of interest.** This process is designed to avoid the kinds of difficulties that can arise when an investigator has a direct economic interest in the outcome of the study to be performed, such as holding stock in a company that produces a particular medication or serving on a salaried board of directors for the company. Consequently, publications resulting from federally funded research are more likely to provide a balanced view of a topic, including both positive and negative findings. A major downside of Federal funding is that it is highly competitive: There are far more researchers requesting funds than can possibly receive money to do their research. There are far-reaching consequences of this budget crunch: Usually funds go to researchers with well-established track records, in an effort to be certain that the dollars are well spent on researchers who will conduct solid studies and produce publishable results. Funds typically go to studies with high probabilities of being useful, rather than to very unusual or innovative studies which might have great promise but are considered more risky because they use unproven techniques or approaches. Related to this trend, funds typically do not support research into treatments for what are known popularly as "orphan diseases." These are rare diseases that affect only a small proportion of people—so research dollars spent to investigate them do not yield the greatest bang for the buck. Consequently, a problem such as Gilles de la Tourette syndrome, a disease with life damaging tics and bizarre behavioral manifestations, remains poorly funded and minimally researched. Typically, funds are not received by investigators who want to replicate already existing research. Considering these funding trends, it is easy to see how research supported by federal agencies can get bogged down in the status quo and can fail to encourage creative efforts on the part of new investigators.

Private foundations span a wide range of funding sources; and a wide range of caveats go along with this diversity. Some private foundations have been established to provide financial support for study of particular issues or diseases, such as research on the prevention/eradication of breast cancer. These private foundations often have been established in the name or memory of someone who has been a victim of the disease targeted by the foundation. The kinds of research projects that are funded depend on the scope of interest of the particular foundation, as does the amount of funding available. There are other private foundations that actually are branches of companies which have been set up to serve the dual functions of tax shelters and philanthropy. Such foundations typically have a somewhat broader scope of interest, such as children's health or enhancing education. Private funding agencies often mirror some of the procedures and requirements set by federal agencies, such as adopting a conflict-of-interest policy. On the other hand, they typically provide smaller funding packages than federal agencies and may be suited to different kinds of studies. However, the broad range of diversity that exists among private foundations makes it useful to find out about a specific foundation's aims and policies when evaluating the research it has supported.

Finally, it is helpful to know that funding sources dole out monies in two basic forms: grants and contracts. The major difference between these two is that grants typically are given to an investigator to perform research which the investigator has proposed doing, while contracts pay the investigator to do work which the funding source wants done. This distinction might seem elusive, but it is important. Both grants and contracts reflect the priorities and values associated with a funding source. However, contracts more clearly provide an environment in which the investigators are "working for" the funding agency to perform a task that has been defined in rather great detail. Grants, on the other hand, typically provide more flexibility for investigators to pursue their proposed goals.

The Anatomy of Medical Investigations

■THE CONCEPT OF DESIGN

To understand the notion of research design, it may be helpful to borrow some ideas from the field of architecture. When plans are drawn up for a building, all essential aspects of the structure are thought through in detail, to be certain that the product will be satisfactorily strong and aesthetically pleasing. When we design a study, a great deal of forethought should be involved to ensure that the product will be robust and elegant. The robustness of a study is the strength of its findings; its elegance is the aesthetically pleasing quality of a study that has been designed with a clarity of focus and an appropriateness of methodology. As an architectural structure is not reducible to the timber, stone, or mortar that have been used to build it, neither is a study reducible to its statistical analysis, sample size, or procedures. Like a building, a research study must be evaluated as a whole. However, if any of its parts are weak, the study will be flawed. If crucial parts are very weak, it will be useless.

One of the most common mistakes made by research consumers is confusing research design with statistical analysis, and thinking that these two concepts are the same. A better way to think about these concepts is that the design of a study will dictate whether statistical analyses are needed and, if so, will suggest the kinds of statistical analyses that should be used. On the other hand, statistical analyses are often a weak link in a study's structure—so, savvy consumers will read the mathematical as well as the nonmathematical parts of an article.

Good research design requires that a study be tied to "reality" on both ends. This means that a good study begins by asking a question (or stating an hypothesis) and ends by answering the same question (supporting or not supporting the hypothesis). Everything that happens in between these points must be done to get from the question to the answer in the best way possible. It is inappropriate to select statistical analyses, methods, or procedures using any other criterion except that of finding the best bridge between the points. So, deciding that you are committed to using a particular statistical analysis and finding yourself in the position of having a statistical method in search of a research question is a wrong-headed way to design research. Similarly, deciding that you must address a particular research question, even though your resources permit you to perform only an inadequate investigation of the topic, is irresponsible research.

■THE BUILDING BLOCKS OF RESEARCH DESIGN

Most good quality research articles provide information about six fundamental building blocks that are thought through during planning phases of the investigation, and which can be reported in detail after the investigation has been completed. These are:

1. Research questions or hypotheses (may also be called objectives or purpose)
2. Rationale for the study
3. Methods
4. Analyses
5. Results
6. Conclusions (and discussion)

Not all research reports will have these sections clearly labeled, and some kinds of research, such as qualitative studies, will not follow precisely the same structure. (Some comments on qualitative research are provided at the end of this chapter.) However, knowing the fundamental building blocks of "classic" studies will assist the research consumer in making a preliminary determination about the adequacy of a piece of research.

Research Questions and Hypotheses

Clearly articulated questions and/or hypotheses inform the reader about the precise purpose of a research study. The title of the article should provide some good clues and an abstract, if one exists, also should help focus the research problem. Typically, some sort of introductory section will precede the specific research questions or hypotheses, so these tend to be included at the end of several paragraphs of text.

Hint: When evaluating this part of a study, ask yourself the following questions.

1. Can I clearly identify the research questions or hypotheses as separate parts of the document—or do I need to "assume" that some unclear statements in text comprise the focus of the research? In other words, have the investigators done their job, or am I forced to formulate the questions/hypotheses myself?
2. Are questions or hypotheses very specific to the study I am reading—or are they so general that they could apply to a vast array of studies? For example, a research question that asks, "Can the clinical course of HIV disease be altered?" is not as helpful as a question that asks more specifically, "Are antiretroviral therapies use-

ful in increasing survival and slowing disease progression in patients with HIV disease?"

3. Are research questions or hypotheses articulated in such a way that they can be addressed by the research that has been performed? For example, a research hypothesis might be stated as, "Antiretroviral therapies increase long-term survival of patients with HIV disease." However, the design of the study has provided for only two months of follow-up. Regardless of the findings of the study, they cannot constitute an adequate response to the long-term aspects of the hypothesis as stated. A preferable restatement might be, "A positive impact of antiretroviral therapy on progression of HIV disease will be seen during a two-month period of study."

Rationale for the Study

This should be a clear statement about why the study has been performed. It often takes the form of several paragraphs that review briefly the state of the art on the particular topic, making some reference to classic studies in the area as well as the most recent relevant research. The rationale should provide the feel of a convincing argument for why time, effort, and money have been spent on this particular piece of research.

Hint: To evaluate this building block, consider the questions that follow.

1. Can I identify a clear rationale for this study? While I expect to read a bit about the research history leading up to this study, I don't want to get bogged down in issues that are peripheral to the topic. How well have the investigators honed down the rationale so that it is obviously a rationale?

2. Am I convinced that this research should have been done/needed to be done? Here, do not get thrown off by studies that are replications. Replications can be enormously helpful to be certain that what has been found by one investigator is "real" and not simply specific to that

investigator's skills, hospital, patients, etc. Consequently, just because it has been done before does not
make a study unnecessary. On the other hand, even ra-
tionales for replications should provide a sense of the
importance of performing the study.

3. Does the rationale give me a sense of where this study
"fits" in terms of the impact it will have on medical care?
For example, what is the role of a re-analysis of TB contagion data from the early part of this century? Does the
rationale provide a clear sense of how results of this re-
analysis will impact on current health care policy and
surveillance procedures; or does it appear to be something of historical interest that is not intended to impact
on contemporary medical practice?

4. Given the present-day information explosion, has the rationale done its job of convincing me to continue reading
this research report—or have I decided that there are
better ways to spend my limited reading hours?

Methods

**The central point of providing a discussion of methods is to
enable other researchers to replicate the study almost exactly.** This section has strong origins in experimental/labora-
tory research, in which everything down to the specific models
of the equipment that was used was spelled out for other investigators. Even if you are not reading a research report with the
intent of replicating the study, this section should provide sufficiently detailed information to help you determine the extent to
which the findings can be generalized to patients other than
those enrolled in the study.

Hint: Ask yourself some questions about how much the
investigators actually have told you.

1. If I did want to replicate this research, do I have enough
information to permit me to do so?

2. Do I know specifically how patients were enrolled in the
study? In other words, do I know not only about the ideal

procedures that were set out in advance, but also about the things that failed to work? If study participation was initially offered to 1000 patients, but only 200 completed the trial, what accounts for the difference in numbers? Did some patients decide to refuse right from the start—and for what reasons? Did others begin to participate and then drop out—and for what reasons?

3. How did the investigator manage patients who responded poorly to a treatment or experienced unacceptable side effects? Were these patients "crossed over" to another group, or simply dropped from the study? If they were "crossed over," how did their results get analyzed (as part of the first group, the second group, or separated out as a third group)?

4. Do I know enough about method of sampling to obtain a good demographic picture? For example, if different ethnicities, ages, genders, geographic locations, etc. might impact on the results of the study, have I been given sufficient information about how these demographic variables were incorporated into the sampling scheme?

5. Do I know specifically how a treatment was administered and/or how assessments of efficacy were done? For example, in a study designed to reduce or eliminate TB, has the investigator provided specific information about whether patients received directly observed therapy (DOT) or whether they were given a prescription to take on their own? Similarly, do I know who provided the care—nurses, medical students, senior physicians, etc.?

6. Do I know specifically which treatment was administered? For example, in studies of the efficacy of bacillus Calmette-Guérin (BCG) vaccine, many different strains of the vaccine have been used—and individual studies have reported efficacies of BCG ranging from zero to 100%. Does the investigator tell me specifically which strain of vaccine, or which form of a medication, was administered, and over what period of time?

The questions that can be raised about Methods are as diverse as the kinds of studies one encounters in the medical literature. However, if you are guided by question number one above, and follow with questions about sampling and procedures, you will have a fairly good sense of how much the researchers have revealed about their methods and how much remains unknown to the consumer.

Analyses

In many studies, this section refers to the statistical analyses that have been performed on the data that have been collected. Often, analyses are not separated from the section on Results, especially if the analyses that have been done are analyses that are typically used for the particular type of study. For example, experimental designs lend themselves to statistical analysis of variance. If analysis of variance has been performed on the data, brief mention of the statistical methods may accompany the Results. On the other hand, if unusual forms of analysis have been used, or analyses are likely to be unfamiliar to most readers, then a more detailed section is necessary. For example, studies using decision analysis continue to incorporate separate sections on the structure and analysis of the decision model.

Hint: Even without an expert grasp of statistical and other methods of analysis, you can determine much about the adequacy of this section of a study with a set of rather general questions.

1. Has the investigator stated specifically which analyses were performed? If the analyses are not indicated by name, there is a major problem with the study.
2. Has the investigator provided a reason for using the particular analyses? If the analyses are ones that would be "expected" given the nature of the study, there is not much need for an explanation. However, if the analyses are atypical, then it is important for the investigator to let

research consumers know what thinking contributed to the choice of analyses.

3. Is there so much statistical jargon that I cannot "translate" the analyses into English? A research report should be written with the assumption that not every reader will be an expert in analytic methods. The job of the investigator is not to teach statistics; but the job of the investigator is to make every part of the research report understandable. Consequently, be wary of studies that seem to be buried in jargon—the jargon might be hiding some messy data or unfounded procedures.

4. Does the investigator mention anything about data not fitting the assumptions of the statistical analyses that were performed? Other ways this point might enter an article is through mention of "transforming data" or "normalizing data." What this means is that something artificial was done to make the data fit the statistical analysis, instead of using an analysis that fits the data. Sometimes such data transformations are helpful and appropriate. Sometimes they lead to deceptive or incorrect results. If an article that is important to your healthcare practice or your own research contains such topics, and you do not understand what has been done, consult an expert who knows both statistics and the general content area that was studied.

5. Do I need help making sense of this section of the article? If you feel insecure about your understanding of the analyses in an important study, by all means seek help from an appropriate consultant. However, be aware that many statisticians, biostatisticians, computer programmers, and mathematicians may not know enough about your content area to help you make an "English translation" from the section on analyses. If you find that your consultant has taught you something about the theories of probability that lie behind curve-fitting, but cannot help you understand how a data transformation might impinge on the results of the study, try to find a consul-

tant who can bridge better the realms of expertise you require.

Results

This section states the results of the analyses as simply and objectively as possible. This is not the place for extrapolations, interpretations, or elaborations. Conclusions and Discussion are intended to serve some of those functions.

It can be quite difficult to determine what fits into Results and what should be held for the Conclusions/Discussion sections of an article. A good rule of thumb is that anything under the rubric of Results should remain within the specific constraints of the analyses that were performed. For example, consider a study in which an analysis was performed to determine whether women with Stage II breast cancer who received adjuvant therapy survived longer than women who did not receive adjuvant therapy. Results might state that there was a statistically significant difference in the lifespans of women who received adjuvant therapy versus those who did not, with a higher lifespan associated with the adjuvant therapy group. Also included in this section would be relevant statistical information, such as the level at which statistical significance had been achieved. What is not appropriate is speculation about what might have happened if the same study had been performed with women diagnosed with Stage III breast cancer. Or, in the case of nonsignificant findings, speculations about why the results were not significantly different.

Hint: The most important questions you can ask yourself about the Results section of an article involve the extent to which you, the research consumer, could literally stop reading at that point and understand how the research questions were answered.

1. Does the Results section, standing without Conclusions and Discussion, enable me to understand what has resulted from this study? In other words, are the findings clearly and readably stated?

2. Is the Results section written in an objective manner, or does it include inappropriate biases on the part of the investigator? In other words, at this point you want to know what happened, not how good or how bad the investigator feels about the results. Be wary of statements such as, "Although the results of this study did not achieve statistical significance, there seems to be a trend toward significance." Typically, this is an attempt to make something out of nothing. (The upcoming statistics section of this chapter, "Unraveling the Misunderstood Roles of Statistics," provides a discussion of the importance—and unimportance—of statistical significance.)

3. If the Results section includes graphic information such as figures, ask yourself if the the graphics help you understand the results. Remember, graphics should be an aid to understanding—not a source of obfuscation.

Conclusions and Discussion

The Results section hopefully has answered the research questions or responded to the hypotheses articulated at the beginning of the report. **The task of the Conclusions and Discussion section(s) primarily is to integrate the results of this study with other findings in the field, particularly with the literature that has been cited in the rationale for the study.** This is also the place where the investigator can indicate the ways in which this study pushes the field forward, advances knowledge, or contributes to better health care. In other words, here is where the investigator may *interpret* the results of the study. However, interpretation must be done scientifically and as objectively as possible.

Hint: Understand that this section may involve some "leaps" beyond what is contained in the Results section. However, such leaps should be made with care and should be labeled as extrapolations or interpretations. Following are some questions that will assist you in making responsible use of the last sections of a research report.

1. Am I relying solely on the investigator's interpretation of the results in order to make sense of this study, or have I also drawn my own conclusions from the Results section? You will benefit most by drawing your own conclusions and comparing them with what you find in the investigator's writing. Inconsistencies between the two can alert you to points you might not have understood well—as well as to points on which the investigator might reveal personal bias.

2. Do the investigator's conclusions follow from the Results? For example, if no differences were found between an experimental and a control group, the conclusions should state this lack of difference. It should not be couched in terms that encourage the reader to assume that a difference does, in fact, exist but was difficult to "see" for some reason.

3. Do the Conclusions and Discussion remain close to the original research question/hypothesis? Or does this section explore tangents that confuse the "answers" to the original question?

4. How well does the investigator integrate the Results of this study with existing work in the field, which should have been cited at the start of the report? The Conclusions and Discussion should assist the reader to understand how the present study fits or fails to fit with expectations derived from previous studies and/or theories.

5. Do the Conclusions and Discussion read like a "position piece" with the investigator standing on a soapbox to sell the findings? If so, go back to the Results and draw your own conclusions.

When time to read research reports is scarce, it is tempting to jump from research questions to conclusions, permitting the investigator to do the job of interpretation. However, it is safest to do the interpreting yourself, based on a thorough reading of the entire article. You may be surprised at how often an investigator's interpretation will differ from your own.

■CLINICAL VERSUS BENCH RESEARCH

In the world of medical investigations, clinical research typically refers to research performed with living human subjects, while "bench" research refers to research performed in chemistry or biology laboratories using cells, viruses, genes, chemicals, etc., rather than the entire human organism. While contrasts exist between these two general types of research, it is important to remember that bench research and clinical research comprise a kind of **research continuum.** Many investigations must begin as bench research before they can lead to large-scale clinical investigations. In fact, the practice of performing Phase I, Phase II, and Phase III trials refers to a continuum in which successful laboratory research (Phase I) must precede research with human participants, and large-scale human trials (Phase III) can follow only successful small-scale trials with human participants who have not responded to existing treatments and are most likely to benefit from a new therapy or procedure (Phase II).

Detractors of bench research argue that models developed from using parts of humans, such as cancer cells or genes, or from using nonhuman animals do not necessarily mimic the responses that would be obtained if the research were conducted with human participants. This is a valid criticism because generalizations cannot be made from cell to person, or from laboratory rat to human. On the other hand, an absence of bench research would mean that all trials would be performed immediately on human participants, without an initial opportunity to work out possible problems. Additionally, work with humans cannot always be conducted under strict experimental conditions. Humans often are studied in what might be considered our "natural habitats." The term "free living" populations refers to investigations in the natural environment, in contrast to quar-

TABLE 3a CLINICAL VERSUS BENCH RESEARCH

Issue	Clinical Research	Bench Research
Research subject	Living human	Human organic matter; nonhuman animals
Research design	Difficult to control, especially in free-living human participants	High degree of experimental control possible
Ethical issues	Typically focus is on the impact on individual human lives	Might be on animal rights; also might involve more global ethical questions such as the impact of genetic engineering

antined or otherwise isolated situations. Table 3a summarizes the major differences between clinical and bench research.

■PROSPECTIVE VERSUS RETROSPECTIVE STUDIES

Many studies in clinical medicine are designed to investigate the course of a disease under varying conditions, perhaps with the intent to find out whether a treatment option or a diagnostic finding has made a difference in the life expectancies or quality of life of patients. Such studies often require that patients be followed for a substantial amount of time. For example, a number of researchers have attempted to answer the question, "Does a finding of lobular carcinoma in situ (LCIS) of the breast predispose a woman to develop invasive breast cancer?" In order to answer this question, women with LCIS must be followed over a number of years, perhaps decades. A study designed to track women for only a few months would not provide an adequate time frame to answer the research question, since most cancers that occur in women diagnosed with LCIS occur years rather than months after LCIS has been diagnosed.

Studies that require long periods of time to perform are costly as well as difficult to perform. Ideally, investigators would decide to develop a **prospective database** comprised of all cases of LCIS that are reported within a well-defined sample of women. Once a woman has been diagnosed with LCIS, all subsequent data that might be relevant to breast disease would be entered into the database. These data might include a broad array of variables, such as the start of hormone replacement therapy or diagnosis of gynecological problems. This is an awesome task to perform, and it is not easily performed by a single investigator. The State of Connecticut Board of Health set up a database called the Connecticut Tumor Registry for the express purpose of prospectively studying women with LCIS. In Connecticut, all tumors are "reportable" findings, meaning that all hospitals and all physicians must provide the Board of Health with data about tumors that have been diagnosed or treated. Consequently, with the exception of women who relocate out of state, women with LCIS are followed in careful detail. Since data also are available on relocation, it is possible to correct the estimates of invasive cancer for numbers of cases lost to follow-up. The resulting information can be used to provide a valid estimate of the likelihood that women from a particular geographic area diagnosed with LCIS will develop invasive breast cancer.

Now, consider the problems that would characterize **retrospective investigations** on the same topic. Retrospective means "looking backward," and that is how retrospective studies function. Most often, retrospective studies involve looking backward into existing medical records. In retrospective studies of LCIS, investigators sifted through patient files to find women who had been diagnosed with this finding at a particular hospital. They used data contained in these patients' files to determine whether a diagnosis of invasive breast cancer had also been entered at some point after the diagnosis of LCIS had been made.

What are the weaknesses of a retrospective approach? Perhaps of greatest importance is the fact that the investigator is not in control of patient follow-up. He or she must take what is available in hospital records or whichever other kind of database is used. And quite frequently, such records are poor or incomplete for the purposes of research because they were not designed to address the specific research question.

In the case of retrospective studies of LCIS, it is possible that a woman diagnosed with LCIS at one hospital did not return to the same hospital when she was diagnosed later with invasive breast cancer. Thus, the investigator would be led to the mistaken conclusion that this woman did not develop invasive breast cancer, and would underestimate risk. Consider also another possible route for error: Women who were diagnosed with LCIS at a different institution came to the study-site hospital for later diagnostic screening and possible treatment of invasive cancer. Their earlier diagnosis of LCIS might never have found its way into the second hospital's records. Finally, the most dramatic cause of systematic bias could be that the reason women had hospital records at all is because they had invasive breast cancer. The finding of LCIS could have been picked up during the medical history. This means that if LCIS were equally distributed among women who do develop invasive breast cancer and those who do not, say at a hypothetical 50% rate, the retrospective study would "see" the "marker" of LCIS present in half of the hospital recorded cases, making LCIS appear falsely to be a strong marker for invasive disease. In all the above scenarios, retrospective study would result either in underestimates or overestimates of risk of invasive cancer associated with LCIS. One of the major weaknesses of retrospective research is that the investigator cannot distinguish between what is a confounding effect of missing data versus what truly is the absence of disease in a particular case. For example: Has a woman investigated through data available at site one truly remained free of invasive breast cancer for the remainder of her life, or did she seek diagnosis and treatment for an invasive lesion at another site that was not linked to her hospital record at site one?

Retrospective designs also have been used to study the impact of medical interventions on patient health. At one urban hospital, a physician in charge of treating asthma patients had initiated a patient education program that he believed would convince patients to comply with their medical regimens and, thus, prevent serious attacks. After the patient education program had been in place for nearly 2 years, the physician decided to perform a retrospective study to determine whether the education program had effectively reduced asthma attacks in patients who had participated in the program. To accomplish this, he located charts for all patients who had received the intervention and checked for information about whether they subsequently had been admitted to the emergency room for asthma attacks. What is flawed in this design? Patients suffering from an acute asthma attack might not come to the same hospital where they had received treatment, particularly if they were some distance away from that hospital when the attack occurred. An acute asthma attack can be a life-threatening situation, requiring patients to seek assistance at the closest possible health center. Without a prospective design that could incorporate other ways of knowing whether patients had experienced acute attacks, such as contacting patients for information from time to time or expanding data collection to health centers state-wide, gross errors can be made. In this case, the investigator found relatively few admissions at his hospital for asthma attacks in his patients, and concluded incorrectly that the educational intervention had prevented acute episodes!

Specific Research Designs for Clinical Studies...................

■THE PERVASIVE PROBLEM OF TIME

Temporal variables create problems for many clinical studies, whether they are strict clinical trials or less rigorous designs. The crux of the problems is that often there is no way to know when a patient initially contracted a disease or to determine whether identifying a disease earlier actually makes a difference in its clinical course.

Prevention and control of tuberculosis provides a contemporary example of the problem of not knowing when an infection was contracted. Tuberculosis is a two-stage process. First, an individual must become infected with the tubercle bacillus. This initial infection is not what most people think of as "TB," because it is not contagious and does not cause symptoms. After this initial infection, there is some likelihood that the individual will develop active tuberculosis during the next few decades. Active TB is what most people think of as tuberculosis: a contagious pulmonary disease characterized by coughing and fever. However, after initial infection, there is a much greater likelihood that the individual will not develop active disease. The strong likelihood that an infected individual will not develop active disease reflects the fact that in most individuals tuberculosis remains essentially dormant.

If a patient has had regular (e.g., yearly) skin testing (Mantoux test) to determine if they are infected with TB, have repeatedly shown negative skin test results, and then suddenly show a positive result after contact with a known case of active tuberculosis, determining the time of infection is relatively straightforward. The patient most likely became infected during the past year. However, this is not how most cases of tuberculosis infection come to the attention of physicians. Since the initial infection is asymptomatic, if it is discovered at all, the discovery typically is made during a routine physical examination, such as a pre-employment physical requiring a tuberculin skin test. With no known active contacts and no regular skin testing, the patient might have become infected within the very recent past or decades ago. Does this matter? Yes, because the risk of developing active tuberculosis from the dormant infection and the argument for using preventive therapy are strongest in the first five years after infection. Without knowing time of infection, not only is it impossible to determine the risk facing the patient, but it is also impossible to determine precisely how well preventive therapy performs because the "baseline" risk for active TB at the time preventive therapy begins is unknown. So, research on preventive therapy for TB can be confounded by an unanswerable question that goes something like this: Has preventive therapy reduced an individual's risk from 10% to zero, or from 2% to zero?

Consider the following example. The physician sees the patient in year 2001, corresponding to point 2 in Figure 3b. If the patient's inital infection occurred in year 2001, his/her risk of developing active TB is estimated at 10% (for otherwise healthy, nonimmune compromised persons). However, suppose that the patient's initial infection occurred 10 years ago, in 1991, corresponding to point 1 in Figure 3b. Given the mathematical curves that are used to estimate risk of developing active TB after inital infection, the patient's risk in 2001 would be lower than 10%. The curves presently in use suggest that the greatest risk of developing active TB, occurs during the first several years after infection, with the remaining risk spread over the patient's lifespan. Since the physician *does not know* when this patient intially was infected, the best estimate suggested for use in determining risk of active TB is 2%. There is no way to know whether the patient is in fact at a higher risk, even as high as 10%.

Consider another temporal problem: the issue of whether diagnosing a disease earlier impacts on our ability to alter its clinical course. One of the procedures that continues to draw some debate along these lines is mammography. It has been documented that the combination of mammography and physical exam identifies more breast cancer lesions, and lesions at earlier stages, than can be detected by physical exam alone. Women who are diagnosed earlier receive treatment earlier in the course of their disease. Does this earlier treatment actually affect life expectancy? There are two vantage points from which this question can be approached. First, it seems reasonable to assume that if effective therapies exist, then treating breast

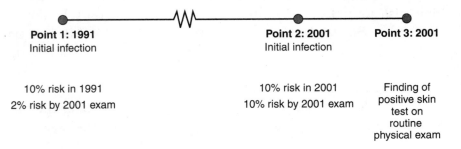

Figure 3b Time problem in assessing risk of active TB.

cancers earlier would more likely result in extensions of life. On the other hand, how do we know that earlier treatment is, in fact, responsible for what appears to be a longer lifespan. Perhaps we have simply "seen" the problem earlier, and so the time from diagnosis to death "looks" longer than it would have if we diagnosed the disease in its later stages. Perhaps all we are doing is looking at a disease from two different points in time, and being deceived into believing that it is not a difference in perspective but rather a true impact on life expectancy that we are seeing.

Figures 3c and 3d show two situations in which the only thing that changes is the time at which we "see" a disease process. This is an illustration of what is known as a **lead time bias.** Figure 3c shows how a diagnostician can be "fooled" into thinking that early detection has resulted in an eight-year extension of life. Figure 3d shows an actual impact of five additional years of life related to early detection.

These temporal issues can become even more complicated when research participants are enrolled in a study sequentially—meaning not all at once—and are followed for varying periods of time. Making good estimates of time to active or invasive disease, or time to mortality, often hinges on the extent to which we have

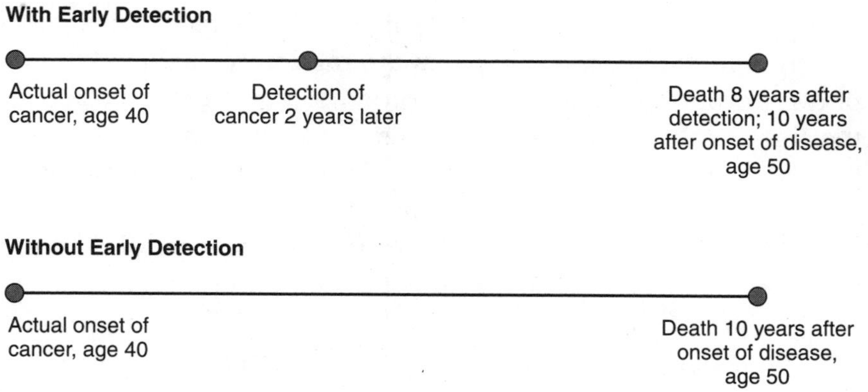

With Early Detection

Actual onset of cancer, age 40	Detection of cancer 2 years later	Death 8 years after detection; 10 years after onset of disease, age 50

Without Early Detection

Actual onset of cancer, age 40	Death 10 years after onset of disease, age 50

Figure 3c Lead time bias.

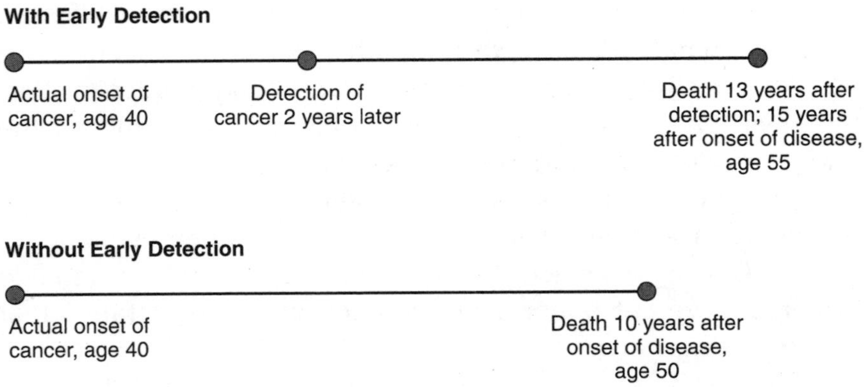

With Early Detection

Actual onset of
cancer, age 40

Detection of
cancer 2 years later

Death 13 years after
detection; 15 years
after onset of disease,
age 55

Without Early Detection

Actual onset of
cancer, age 40

Death 10 years after
onset of disease,
age 50

Figure 3d Actual impact.

good estimates of the onset of disease or infection. And making good estimates of the efficacies of therapies often hinges on the extent to which we can be sure that our findings are not merely the expression of some kind of temporal bias.

■CLINICAL TRIAL METHODOLOGY

Clinical trial methodology is clinical medicine's version of classic experimental design. However, in clinical trials, the study is done using human participants, rather than cells, viruses, laboratory rats, or other nonhuman "subjects." In clinical trials, as in experimental design, participants are **randomly assigned** to one of two or more groups. The experimenter exercises control over the treatments each group receives. This might mean that one groups gets a true treatment (an intervention of some sort) while another group serves as a control (no actual intervention). A true experiment might also mean that several different treatments are being compared with each other, so that for example, group A gets intervention #1, group B gets intervention #2, and group C gets intervention #3. The important points are: There is always more than one group, so that a basis exists for comparison; and the groups are as equivalent as possible with respect to everything except the intervention(s).

A generic example of clinical trial methodology is shown schematically in Figure 3e. This example includes a control group, C, with participants who receive no medical intervention, as well as two treatment groups, A and B, with participants who receive two different kinds of medical intervention. All participants are randomly assigned to one of the three groups. Evaluation means that the patients are assessed for the degree of their illness both before and after the intervention period, regardless of whether they have received one of the interventions or have participated as a member of the control group. From this generic structure, it should be clear that clinical trials are prospective studies.

Why is a basis of comparison needed in clinical trials? Suppose an investigator claims finally to have found a cure for the common cold. The investigator's research consists of only one group of patients, all of whom have sought treatment for colds. The investigator prescribed oral antibiotics for the patients and instructed them to return in 2 weeks for reevaluation. After 2 weeks, all patients' colds were gone. Did the antibiotic

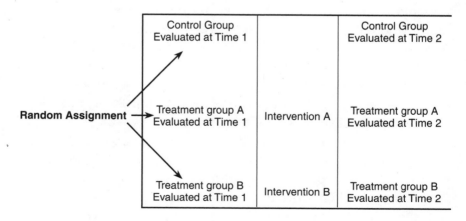

Figure 3e Generic structure of clinical trial methodology.

cure the colds? It is not possible to know, because people with colds who did not take antibiotics might also have been "cured" within 2 weeks, simply because most common colds run a natural course of less than that amount of time.

Now consider an alternative scenario: Suppose the patients who came for treatment all returned in 2 weeks still feeling miserably symptomatic, in spite of the fact that they had all been on antibiotic therapy. Can the physician conclude that antibiotic therapy is useless for treating colds? No, because there was no basis for comparison. Perhaps without antibiotics, these particular patients might have become more seriously ill; perhaps their colds would have progressed to bacterial pneumonia if they had not had antibiotic therapy. Such a conjecture is plausible because most people do not seek physician intervention for common colds, so patients who visit a physician for a cold might be more ill than those who do not.

In this example, the need for a basis of comparison is clear. What about random assignment to a treatment (e.g., antibiotic) and a control (e.g., no antibiotic) group? In order to have a scientific basis for making claims about the effects of antibiotic therapy, it is crucial to be as certain as possible that those patients receiving therapy are similar to those without therapy. Consequently, it would not be sound scientifically to compare patients who came to a physician requesting treatment to patients who did not bother to seek treatment for their colds. The very fact that one group sought intervention suggests that they are "different" from the group that took care of their colds themselves. Perhaps those who visited a physician were more ill, as suggested above, or perhaps they had histories of serious respiratory disease, perhaps they were elderly—or young children—and more at risk than the rest of the population, or perhaps they were simply more conscientious about taking care of their health. Perhaps those who did not visit a physician were so ill that they could not get to a health center, perhaps they could not afford a physician visit, or perhaps they were "veterans" of colds who know they wind up feeling better after 3 days regardless of what they do. All of the above factors could impact on the outcomes of treatment, and create deceptive results that might appear either to favor or disfavor the use of antibiotic therapy.

In addition to the structure of clinical trials illustrated above, the specific methods used in conducting the study are important to consider. Of great importance are the practices of blinding and double-blinding. **Blinding** means that participants in a study are not told which group they are in while the study is being run. The informed consent form, which they would have been required to sign, would have informed them that they might receive an actual treatment for their illness or a "placebo." A **placebo** is something that resembles treatment, such as a pill containing only inert ingredients, which ensures that participants do not know that they are in a control group. Blinding is particularly important when patients' reports of symptoms and side effects serve as measures of the efficacy of treatments. Patients who know they are on a treatment regimen might be more likely to expect side effects, and to expect to feel better, than those who know they are receiving no treatment for their illness. Such expectations can exert an unconscious bias and impact on patients' reports of their progress. **Double-blinding** means that not only the participants but also the investigators, or the physicians who are evaluating the patients in the trial, are deprived of knowledge about which patients are in which groups. Keeping the investigators/physicians blind to group membership helps ensure that they will not see "what they want to see" or "what they expect to see" when they evaluate patient progress. In other words, both blinding and double-blinding help minimize the effects of bias on study outcomes.

Sometimes research questions require that more than one health care site be involved in an investigation. This is the case when the investigation focuses on treatment options for a rare disease, such as a rare form of cancer, which might be diagnosed only a few times each year at a single site. When clinical trial methodology is expanded to involve more than one site, it is known as a **multicenter trial.** In multicenter trials, great care must be taken to ensure that patients who are enrolled in the study groups are equivalent to each other on all important factors, and that the methods used to dispense treatment and obtain evaluations are standardized across sites. In other words, great care must be taken to maintain the rigorous standards of clinical trial methodology in light of the fact that using more than one study site can present sources of undesirable variability, also known as "error."

There are many reasons why good clinical trials are relatively rare in medical research. These reasons include the ethical dilemmas involved in depriving patients of knowledge about whether they are receiving treatment, as well as the costs of performing good trials. On the other hand, solid clinical trial methodology permits researchers to get as close as possible to establishing cause-and-effect relations between treatment options and health outcomes. Studies that depart in any way from strict clinical trial methodology do not permit researchers to make statements which suggest that doing something (such as providing a particular treatment) results in a particular outcome (such as curing a disease).

■COHORT STUDIES

Under some conditions, it is unethical to randomly assign participants to "intervention" groups, particularly when the intervention is an exposure to a negative or damaging condition. For example, an investigator might ask the question, "How does exposure to HIV disease in utero affect the psychomotor development of infants?" Ethically the investigator cannot selectively expose some fetuses to HIV disease and spare others. However, to understand the possible impact of HIV exposure on infants' development, the investigator requires a basis of comparison.

One possible approach to this question is through analysis of a **cohort** of infants, some of which have been exposed to HIV and some of which have not. An investigator might seek to enroll in the study a sample of mothers including those who are HIV-seropositive and those who are HIV-seronegative. After the infants are born and sufficient time has elapsed to establish serostatus, they will be classified into three groups: HIV-seronegative child from HIV-seronegative mother; HIV-seronegative child from HIV-seropositive mother; and HIV-seropositive child from HIV-seropositive mother. The infants will be followed for a period of time sufficient to permit differences in psychomotor development to emerge if they do, in fact, exist. Infants will be tested at selected time intervals to make an assessment of psychomotor development. A schematic view of this study is shown in Figure 3f.

From this illustration, it can be seen that like clinical trials, cohort studies are prospective. They begin at a point in time and move forward into the future. What is different from clinical trials is that there is no randomization, and the investigator does not exercise control over the intervention or exposure. Furthermore, participants in a cohort study are not "blinded" to their group membership. Because participants are not blinded, it is difficult if not impossible to blind investigators/physicians to the group memberships of the cohort. This is because discussion of the participants' health and treatment is likely to comprise a

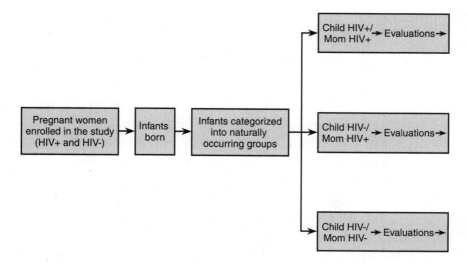

Figure 3f Example of a cohort study.

significant part of the interaction that occurs between participant and physician, in this example between mothers and pediatricians.

Cohort studies are clinical medicine's version of what is
known in other fields as **longitudinal studies.** Longitudinal studies typically follow participants over relatively lengthy periods
of time and involve multiple assessments, in contrast to performing only one assessment, or performing more than one assessment within a short time frame, such as a period of weeks.

One of the advantages of cohort studies is that they provide
a view of "real life." In other words, they are not distorted by strict
experimental conditions but rather reflect the natural unfolding of
a particular disease or exposure. On the other hand, cohort studies do not lend themselves to making causal statements. In the
example above, suppose that HIV+ children show delays in psychomotor development that are not exhibited by the two HIV-
groups. Is it exposure to HIV disease that causes developmental
delays? Or is it that HIV+ infants spend more time in hospital set-
tings, and have less opportunity to exercise psychomotor skills?
These questions highlight the fact that when the rigorous control
associated with clinical trial methodology is impossible, it is also
impossible to make causal statements about interventions (or ex-
posures) and their outcomes.

Like clinical trials, cohort studies can involve a great deal
of expense, much of which comes from the amount of person-
power required to keep in touch with a free-living study population. One of the most troublesome sources of error in cohort
studies is the number of participants who are lost to follow-up.
When individuals cease to participate, it is important for the investigator to attempt to find out why they have terminated their
participation and to report the reasons. A critical question for
the research consumer to ask about this loss, also known as **attrition,** is whether more participants have dropped out of one
group than out of the others. This is known as **differential attrition,** and can result in extremely distorted findings. In the HIV
infant example, suppose that 50% of the HIV+ children have
been lost to follow-up after 2 years. The remaining HIV+ chil-

dren show no differences in development when compared with the HIV– children (who have only a 2% attrition). Does this finding reveal that no developmental differences exist between HIV+ and HIV– children after 2 years of age? Or has something else happened here? Perhaps the HIV+ children who were lost to follow-up were significantly more ill than those who continued in the study. Perhaps if the HIV+ children who were lost to follow-up had been evaluated at 2 years old, they would have shown significant developmental delays when compared with the HIV– groups. The point is that once differential attrition has occurred, it is virtually impossible to know how to interpret the results of a cohort study.

Something that can comprise both a strength and a weakness in cohort studies is the fact that every cohort is unique. The developmental psychologists, Baltes and Nesselroade (1979), discussed cohort studies as representing a "unique cultural moment" meaning that the individuals being studied are progressing through a sociopolitical milieau which will never be replicated. Consequently, the investigators may be able to learn a great deal about one cohort of participants, but that knowledge might not generalize to any other cohorts studied at any other times. Studies of periodontal disease, for example, require long time frames to help determine whether particular oral hygiene and dietary habits are correlated with the development of gum disease. Such studies may span decades, during which the sociopolitical milieau will impact on the participants: participants might become more aware of the importance of oral health, perhaps as a result of more intense media coverage of the topic; advertising might intensify its focus on oral health as an important aspect of "sex appeal" or other culturally defined desirables; dietary changes might occur as a result of a culture's growing affluence or increased poverty; new dental procedures and products may become available for treating and/or preventing gum disease. Studies of periodontal disease begun in the 1930s would be quite likely to show different results from similarly designed studies begun in the 1990s. Another dramatic example of the impact of the outside world on investigations is the emergence of available computer technology: It is unlikely that studies designed during the 1970s to track progress in changing medical curricula, such as the impact of problem-based learning versus memorization, could have projected that U.S. medical students would be surfing the Web for vicarious visits to medical databases in Sweden, Great Britain, Japan, etc., to find state-of-the-art answers to their clinical questions!

In order to avoid the possible pitfalls associated with cohort designs, some researchers elect to use **cross-sectional designs.** Instead of following a single cohort over many decades, a cross-sectional study selects participants from each of the time frames of particular interest. In the case of the periodontal studies, an investigator might study adults in each decade of life, e.g., 20-year olds, 30-year olds, 40-year olds, etc., instead of waiting two decades for the 20-year olds to become 40-years old. The problem, of course, is that such cross-sections can provide very different results from longitudinal cohort studies, because in two decades, today's 20-year olds will have traversed a different sociopolitical environment than today's 40-year olds have experienced in the past two decades.

■CASE-CONTROL STUDIES

Case-control studies in clinical medicine are analogous to "known-groups" designs in the social sciences. In known-groups designs, a study begins at the point at which individuals have already fallen into one group or another. Unlike clinical trials, which rely on random assignment to groups, case-controls use naturally occurring groups. One way to understand case-control studies is by contrast with cohort studies. Consider a cohort study designed to answer this question, "Which people in the United States will have heart attacks during their lifetimes?" The investigator will be interested particularly in the variables that will differentiate those who have heart attacks from those who do not. For this example, suppose that the variable of interest is the level of cholesterol in the individual's diet.

To answer the research question using a cohort study, the investigator would need to consider the number of people who have heart attacks each year. In the United States, approximately 1.5 million heart attacks (myocardial infarctions) occur in a population base of approximately 240 million people. This means that there will be approximately one and one-half heart attacks per year for every 240 people enrolled in a cohort study. In order to obtain a sufficient sample of individuals for this cohort study, many thousands of participants would be necessary. This large-scale study might not be feasible for the investigator to perform.

Now, consider how the study would differ if it began with patients known to have had heart attacks, and compared their diets with patients who have not had heart attacks. There are a number of ways in which "control" patients could be obtained. For example, if the case-control study is hospital-based, the investigator might attempt to enroll patients admitted for noncardiac causes to serve as a comparison with those admitted for heart attacks. Another approach would be to draw "controls" from the free-living population in the geographic area from which the heart attack patients were drawn. One important guideline in selecting controls is to be careful that they are not suffering from a related disease, such as coronary artery disease, or have had a heart attack at a previous point in time. On the other hand, the investigator must not exclude controls on the basis of high cholesterol diets: This would be "stacking the decks," and distorting the findings. In other words, the controls should have as likely a chance to have had high cholesterol diets as the cases, if that is the reality of the situation.

Once cases and controls are identified, the investigator attempts to learn as much about the diets of each individual in each group over their lifetimes. This information gathering is clearly looking backward, making case-control studies primarily **retrospective**. Figure 3g provides an illustration of how the sample study might be conceptualized.

As can be seen in Figure 3g, not all cases have high cholesterol diets; and not all controls have low cholesterol diets. In fact,

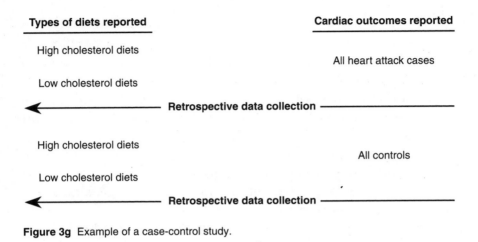

Figure 3g Example of a case-control study.

investigators often are suspicious of findings that are "perfect." In the natural world, it is much more likely that some cases will not have the risk factor or exposure of interest and that some controls will have it. Of course, the expectation of the investigator is that the proportion of cases with the risk/exposure will be greater than the proportion of controls with the risk/exposure.

While case-control studies tend to be more feasible than cohort studies, they are vulnerable to sources of error that can distort the results. One of the most common sources of error lies in the selection of inappropriate controls. Continuing with the heart attack example performed with hospital-based samples, suppose that in order to avoid the error of selecting controls with a diagnosis that might be related to heart disease, the investigator selected patients hospitalized for elective surgeries. How would the results appear if the elective surgery patients were primarily individuals electing arthroscopic procedures for sports injuries? On the other hand, how would the results appear if the elective surgery patients were primarily middle-aged individuals electing gastric bypass surgery for chronic obesity? When compared with the sports-injured arthroscopic patients, the heart attack cases might be likely to report higher cholesterol diets because the athletes who comprise the control group can be expected to be more conscientious about nutrition. On the other hand, the heart attack patients might have consumed less cholesterol than the chronic obesity patients. Neither set of controls truly represents the general population of non-heart attack individuals. Consequently, the study would suffer from **confounding** under either condition.

In addition to the above problem, case-control studies rely heavily on **self-report.** While the use of self-report data is not limited to case-control studies, a large segment of the case-control data is often obtained through interviews with study participants. Self-report data are vulnerable in two ways:

1. Participants must be willing to provide truthful answers;
2. Participants must be able to provide truthful answers.

Being willing means that participants have no reason to lie or to attempt to give the investigator socially desirable answers. In other words, participants must be willing to admit to the investigator (and to themselves!) that they have engaged in the risk behavior/exposure. This posed a major problem in early studies that attempted to identify the risk behaviors associated with HIV disease. Being able to provide accurate data means that the patient must know the answers to the investigator's questions. Studies that ask patients about the kinds of "street" drugs they have used often obtain poor data because even if patients are willing to reveal information, they may not know precisely what was contained in the preparations they used.

The self-report data used in case-control studies becomes less reliable as:

1. The length of recall increases (e.g., from the past two weeks to the past two decades);
2. The complexity of the information increases (e.g., from the prescription medications presently being taken to all prescriptions medications ever taken); and
3. The social undesirability of the topic increases (e.g., from questions about how patients feel about crime to questions about which crimes they have committed).

While case-control studies have inherent weaknesses, they are useful for studying particular types of medical problems, such as rare diseases (that would otherwise require impossibly huge samples) and outbreaks of infections.

TABLE 3b COMPARISON OF STUDY TYPES

	Clinical Trial	Cohort Study	Case-Control
General Type of Design	Experimental	Longitudinal	Known-groups
Time Frame	Prospective, relatively short	Prospective, relatively long	Retrospective
Major Advantages	Reveals causal links	Reveals natural course in free-living participants	Permits study of long-term phenomena in short time span
Major Disadvantages	Ethical constraints experimenting with humans	Losses to follow-up including differential attrition	Confounding in selection of controls; reliance on participant memory of past events
Level of Feasibility	Difficult—Requires exhaustive consideration of patient rights	Difficult—Requires enormous person power to maintain study sample	Less difficult—Requires less time, poses fewer direct threats to physical well-being

■DESIGNS AT A GLANCE

Table 3b provides a summary of the major similarities and differences among clinical trials, cohort studies, and case-control studies.

Unraveling the Misunderstood Roles of Statistics...............

There are three kinds of lies. Lies, damned lies, and statistics.
Benjamin Disraeli

Some people hate the very name of statistics but I find them full of beauty and interest. Whenever they are not brutalized . . . and are warily interpreted, their power of dealing with complicated phenomena is extraordinary.
Francis Galton

■MATHEMATICAL GYMNASTICS

Research consumers often are warned that investigators can lie with statistics and that statistics can be used to make virtually anything look significant. Since both parts of this warning have a basis in reality, it makes sense to begin this section with some general caveats regarding statistics. As you consider these caveats, recall the advice provided earlier in this chapter: **Read all parts of a research report, not just the conclusions and discussion.** You might find that after reading the statistical section, your conclusions differ dramatically from those contained in the report!

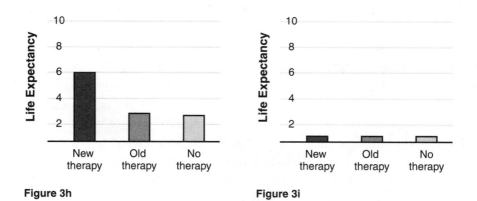

Figure 3h   Figure 3i

First Caveat

Recognize that summary statistics presented in graphic form can be graphed to form just about any conclusion the investigator desires. Consider the different impacts of the following two presentations of results (Figures 3h and 3i).

Data presented in Figure 3h provide a convincing picture of a new therapy which is clearly superior to either the old therapy or no therapy at all. In contrast, data presented in Figure 3i show results of a study in which the differences among a new therapy, an older one and no therapy appear relatively meaningless. Actually, the data presented in both figures reflect the results of the same study: a study of the efficacy of a (hypothetical) new drug, traditional chemotherapy, and no therapy on life expectancies of patients with primary liver cancer. **The difference between the two presentations is that the vertical axis in Figure 3h denotes *months* of life, while the vertical axis in Figure 3i denotes *years* of life.** Consequently, both figures show that patients with primary liver cancer survive less than half a year, regardless of treatment. The difference between the new therapy and other options is approximately 3 months of life.

Hint: When interpreting graphic presentations of data, be sure to look at what comprises the axes because "shrinking" or "blowing up" an axis can create dramatically different effects.

Second Caveat

When one statistical technique fails to work, an investigator may resort to a multitude of statistical methods in an attempt to find meaning in the data. "Do enough tests of statistical significance and you finally will get a significant result through chance alone," says one of the rules of probability.

Be particularly cautious if the statistical tests that were planned at the outset of the study failed to yield statistically significant results and the investigator followed these tests with a series of attempts to fit the results to other statistics. On the other hand, sometimes the statistical tests that were planned rest on assumptions that are not met by the actual data, such as when a "normal distribution" is required in order to perform the statistical test, or when data that are expected to fall along a straight line turn out not to be linear but rather to fall along an S-shaped curve. Such "data realities" actually might turn out to be important findings, so they should not be ignored simply because they were unplanned. But these kinds of findings are different from the approach sometimes called "shotgun empiricism" where anything and everything is tried in an effort to salvage what appear to be meaningless results.

Hint: Look for elegance in the statistical analyses that were performed, just as you look for elegance in the overall design of the study. Elegance in statistical analysis usually means that the researcher has used the most direct route possible to answer the research question, without cluttering the study with a multitude of statistical tests (particularly when the first analysis in the report failed to yield statistically significant results!).

Third Caveat

"If you continue to increase your sample size, at some point you will achieve statistical significance," says another rule of probability. Because our statistical methods come from a tradition in which large sample sizes tend to be valued over small sample sizes, we often tend to overlook the flaw of samples that are too large, expanded beyond the initially planned size, or ridiculously heterogeneous. As is discussed in detail later in this chapter, statistical significance indicates one thing only: the extent to which something that has been found in a study sample is likely to be what the investigator would have found if an entire population rather than a sample had been studied. This has nothing to do with clinical importance, meaningfulness, or value.

Perhaps a study was designed to examine possible differences in patients' responses to traditional hemodialysis versus continuous ambulatory peritoneal dialysis. The primary outcome of interest was level of cognitive functioning, i.e., absence of hepatic encephalopathy. With 30 patients per group, matched on etiology of disease and subject to strict exclusion criteria, no difference was found between the two methods of dialysis. As a result, the investigator continued to enroll additional patients in the study, relaxing criteria in order to obtain as many participants as possible. Patients with histories of psychiatric illness were enrolled, as were patients whose disease etiology was severe trauma, which included closed head injury as well as kidney damage. With 200 patients in each group, differences between the groups reached statistical significance. This study is severely flawed: You are being asked to believe that it is possible to combine apples and oranges, i.e., patients with important differences in etiologies, and to ignore a crucial confounding variable, i.e., other sources of impaired cognition besides the method of dialysis. If the study failed to show differences with samples of 30, why should the reader be convinced that results found with samples of 200 are preferable?

Hint: If a study began with a solid rationale for its sample size, including an explanation of the fact that the size would have enough power to detect whatever the study was designed to uncover, be wary of increased samples that are obtained for no other reason except to attempt to achieve statistical significance.

■DESCRIPTION VERSUS INFERENCE

> I consider the word probability as meaning the state of mind with respect to an assertion, a coming event, or any other matter on which absolute knowledge does not exist.
> August De Morgan

There are two major functions of statistics: to provide quantitative descriptions of research findings and to provide a basis from which the findings of a single study can be generalized to a larger population. These functions differ so dramatically that they comprise two separate subfields of statistics—descriptive and inferential. It is in the realm of inferential statistics that most difficulty arises, because these are techniques designed to deal with uncertainty, particularly to estimate the **probability** that something has occurred and will occur again.

Descriptive statistics usually take the form of frequency counts, percentages, averages (means), and standard deviations. Often they are used to express results of large-scale surveys. For example, data collected by the National Centers for

Disease Control and Prevention (CDC) indicated that as of June 2000, there were 52,873 reported cases of individuals living with AIDS in New York State. Of these, 811 were less than 13 years old. A more full breakdown of geographic locations of persons living with AIDS is shown in Table 3c, which is a segment of a nationwide table generated by the CDC. This table is a good example of how descriptive statistics look. (Survey research as a particular type of design has not been discussed in this chapter on clinical research. It is used largely in the domain of public health research, and so is discussed in Chapter 5, Assessing the Health of Populations.)

When used in large-scale surveys, descriptive statistics make huge amounts of data manageable by providing single "statistics" that express what has happened to many individual cases. The data have been subjected to what is called "data reduction" to make hundreds of thousands of data points understandable in a single number. Results of surveys typically are reported in tables or figures.

Another use of descriptive statistics is to provide information about the characteristics of a study sample so that readers of a research report will be able to determine the extent to which patients in the investigator's sample are similar to the reader's patients. For example, a study of tuberculosis prevention in HIV-seropositive patients might provide descriptive statistics regarding age, gender, ethnicity, and etiology. If the study reports that 100% of its participants were intravenous drug users, a physician who treats HIV-seropositive gay men will know that the study sample is different in some ways from his/her clinic patients—a warning that the rest of the study might not be relevant for this physician's patient clientele.

Survey research often is characterized by a kind of measurement called self-report. Census data, political opinion polls, and market research are commonly encountered nonmedical examples of survey research that relies on self-report.

Inferential statistics are identifiable by the fact that they are associated with what are commonly called "p values," i.e.,

TABLE 3c. PERSONS REPORTED TO BE LIVING WITH HIV INFECTION AND WITH AIDS, BY STATE AND AGE GROUP, REPORTED THROUGH JUNE 2000

Area of Residence (Date HIV Reporting Initiated)	LIVING WITH HIV INFECTION			LIVING WITH AIDS			CUMULATIVE TOTALS		
	Adults/ Adolescents	Children <13 Years Old	Total	Adults/ Adolescents	Children <13 Years Old	Total	Adults/ Adolescents	Children <13 Years Old	Total
Alabama (Jan. 1988)	4,882	40	4,922	2,985	25	3,010	7,867	65	7,932
Alaska (Feb. 1999)	13	–	13	231	1	232	244	1	245
Arizona (Jan. 1987)	4,155	36	4,191	3,064	9	3,073	7,219	45	7,264
Arkansas (July 1989)	1,921	21	1,942	1,535	23	1,558	3,456	44	3,500
California	–	–	–	43,068	218	43,286	43,068	218	43,286
Colorado (Nov. 1985)	5,325	27	5,352	2,806	7	2,815	8,133	34	8,167
Connecticut (July 1992)	–	95	95	5,613	76	5,689	5,613	171	5,784
Delaware	–	–	–	1,123	15	1,138	1,123	15	1,138
District of Columbia	–	–	–	5,962	92	6,054	5,962	92	6054
Florida (July 1997)	16,546	158	16,704	33,643	610	34,253	50,189	768	50,957
Georgia	–	–	–	9,826	93	9,919	9,826	93	9,919
Hawaii	–	–	–	969	5	974	969	5	974
Idaho (June 1986)	294	4	298	219	5	219	513	4	517
Illinois	–	–	–	9,447	134	9,581	9,447	134	9,581
Indiana (July 1988)	3,145	34	3,179	2,575	17	2,592	5,720	51	5,771
Iowa (July 1996)	283	3	286	600	4	604	883	7	890

Kansas (July 1999)	828	11	839	961	5	966	1,789	18	1,806
Kentucky	–	–	–	1,540	15	1,555	1,540	15	1,555
Louisiana (Feb. 1993)	5,587	98	6,785	5,275	55	5,330	11,962	153	12,115
Maine	–	–	–	430	7	437	430	7	437
Maryland	–	–	–	9,352	165	9,517	9,352	165	9,517
Massachusetts	–	–	–	6,538	78	6,613	6,535	78	6,613
Michigan (April 1992)	4,459	93	4,552	4,296	34	4,332	8,757	127	8,884
Minnesota (Oct. 1985)	2,482	28	2,510	1,557	13	1,570	4,039	41	4,080
Mississippi (Aug. 1988)	4,008	47	4,055	1,961	27	1,988	5,969	74	6,043
Missouri (Oct. 1987)	4,136	45	4,181	4,157	17	4,174	8,293	62	8,355
Montana	–	–	–	161	–	161	161	–	161
Nebraska (Sept. 1995)	463	7	470	447	4	451	910	11	921
Nevada (Feb. 1992)	2,574	24	2,598	2,074	11	2,085	4,648	35	4,683
New Hampshire	–	–	–	472	4	476	472	4	476
New Jersey (Jan. 1992)	12,033	372	12,405	14,495	265	14,760	26,528	637	27,165
New Mexico (Jan. 1998)	589	3	802	922	6	928	1,621	9	1,530
New York	–	–	–	52,062	811	52,873	52,062	811	52,873
North Carolina (Feb. 1990)	8,766	110	8,876	4,295	51	4,346	13,061	161	13,222
North Dakota (Jan. 1988)	63	1	64	44	1	45	107	2	109

From Centers for Disease Control and Prevention web site: www.cdc.gov
Note: Complete table not reproduced.

levels of probability usually expressed as statistical significance used or achieved in a study. A level of **statistical significance** indicates that a statistical test has been performed to determine the probability that groups differ from each other or whether variables are related to each other. Some common statistical tests are the t test, F test, Chi square, and Fisher's Z. Information obtained from performing a statistical test enables the researcher to make such statements as: statistically significant differences were found among the groups participating in the clinical trial; or the relation between particular variables such as quality of life and life expectancy was found to be statistically significant.

■STATISTICAL VERSUS CLINICAL SIGNIFICANCE

Inferential statistics and, most importantly the concept of statistical significance, indicate one thing only: **the likelihood that what has been found in a study *sample* would be found if an entire *population* had been studied instead of the sample.** In other words, inferential statistics permit us to study relatively small groups of people and to make inferences about much larger groups. These statistics express the probability that what has been found in a single study reflects larger and/or other populations.

Because statistical significance is a bridge of greater or lesser confidence between a sample and a population, larger samples are more likely than smaller samples to provide reflections of the population. If we wanted to study the comparative effects of beta-blockers versus calcium channel blockers on patients with hypertension, a study that randomly assigned 10,000 people to each group would be more likely to reflect the population of hypertensives than a study that randomly assigned only 10 people to each group. Suppose the study using 10,000 per group found a difference in diastolic blood pressure of 3 points between the groups, and included a statistical test that indicated that this result was statistically significant. The same 3-point difference found in the study of 10 per group is unlikely to be statistically significant when a statistical test is performed. Why would the same difference between groups be statistically significant in one study and not significant in the other? The answer is that statistical significance has virtually nothing to do with clinical importance or the absolute difference between groups. It addresses only the probability that if *all* hypertensives were studied, instead of 20 or 20,000, the results would be similar to those found in the study sample.

Statistical significance is a necessary but not sufficient condition for evaluating the results of a study. Stated simply, if statistical significance is achieved, it provides a degree of confidence that the results of the study are likely to be "real" rather than due purely to chance. On the other hand, it does not tell us whether the results of the study are important. Is a 3-point difference in diastolic blood pressure important? Does it have any clinical relevance, as in helping physicians decide which of two medications to prescribe? The answer clearly is NO—the change in blood pressure is far too small to be clinically important. Consequently, a study can yield results that are statistically significant but clinically insignificant. Thus, attending only to levels of statistical significance is a serious oversight.

In addition to determining whether the results of a study are statistically significant, it is crucial to determine whether they are clinically significant. **Clinical significance** refers to the real-world importance and application of a study's results. If the hypertension study had resulted in a 50-point, statistically significant difference between the groups, this finding would have been both clinically and statistically significant.

Now consider a drastically different scenario. Suppose a study was designed to determine whether a new drug was capable of curing HIV disease. Imagine that the study sample was extremely small: five patients in an untreated control group, and five patients on the new drug protocol. After 6 weeks, one of the patients on the new drug protocol showed no evidence of HIV disease—essentially indicating a cure. Statistical tests performed on these data would not be significant. However, a cure of one patient with HIV disease would constitute one of the greatest milestones in contemporary medicine. This example was provided to suggest that statistical significance be regarded with a healthy degree of skepticism: Very often it is quite important—and sometimes it is not important at all.

■POWER, SAMPLE SIZE, AND TWO TYPES OF ERRORS

In the tonsillectomy example discussed earlier (Bakewin, 1945), the type of error that was made by the physicians who examined the child participants was a "false-positive error." A false-positive means that you conclude something exists when it does not.

The opposite kind of error, a "false-negative error" also occurs in medicine. The practice of obtaining a "second opinion" particularly when surgery is at issue, was prompted by the work of McCarthy (1974). Working as a physician for a trade union, McCarthy demonstrated that when members of the trade union obtained a second opinion before undergoing a range of surgical procedures, approximately 25% obtained negative opinions from the second expert. Most patients heeded the second opinion and opted against surgery. Insurance companies were impressed by this finding, since obtaining a second opinion is significantly cheaper than surgery, and began to implement regulations by which second opinions were required for many medical procedures. Thinking along the lines of the Bakewin (1945) study, one wonders what would have happened to the rate of recommended surgeries if McCarthy had invoked a third or fourth opinion. In the tonsillectomy study, false-positive results were rampant. In the hypothetical extension of the McCarthy study, one wonders what the rate of false negatives would be!

Of course, one of the problems with getting a second opinion is that the second health care provider is being called upon to validate or confirm a condition that has already been labeled as a positive finding, i.e., a medical condition requiring therapeutic action. Second opinions are rarely if ever permitted if the first opinion was negative, i.e., finding no reason for therapeutic action. Consequently, the job of the second opinion expert is to determine whether the finding is truly positive; in other words, to look for negative cases. This orientation can result in a false-negative bias—failing to see something even though it really exists.

These two types of errors, false positives and false negatives, have parallels in research design. If a study is conducted using very small samples, it will be more difficult to achieve statistical significance than if it were conducted on a large sample. This means that the researcher may conclude that nothing has happened: A new treatment has not worked any better than an old treatment, an intervention has not been effective, a promising new diagnostic modality is not as sensitive as was expected, etc. In such instances, the researcher may be making a false-negative error. From a statistical standpoint it may appear that nothing has happened—but that might be because the sample size was too small to achieve statistical significance.

On the other hand, an investigator may have enrolled so many people in a given study's experimental and control groups that even very small (and clinically unimportant) results may yield statistical significance. Thus, the investigator might believe that a new therapy is more efficacious than an old therapy, as in the hypertension example provided earlier, in spite of the fact that the reduction in blood pressure is so small as to be clinically useless. This kind of error in research design and interpretation is a false-positive error.

In order to design studies with sample sizes that are appropriate to detect a desired effect, we can use **power analysis.** In order to determine the target sample size for a study using power analysis, the researcher must know the smallest effect size that is important to detect as well as the desired "power" to detect it. Using the hypertension example, an effect size might be set at a 10-point reduction in diastolic pressure. The researcher will also need to determine how much "detection" power the study should have, ranging from zero power to a power of 100%. If power is set at 80% (a rather typical level) and an effect size is set at 10 points diastolic blood pressure, the study will be said to be 80% likely to detect an effect of 10 points or larger. Also figuring into this equation is the probability level that is set as a cutoff for statistical significance, the convention being .05 or .01. The power to detect an effect is always related to both the size of the effect and the cutoff probability that must be achieved to be labeled "statistically significant."

While power analysis can be helpful in many studies, it can also present problems. First, in many studies in which the size of a clinically meaningful effect is not clearly established, setting an effect size amounts to an educated (and sometimes not so educated) guess. When the desired effect size is not known, power analysis loses its meaning. A different problem emerges when the researcher misunderstands the meaning and use of power analysis, decides that more is always better, and greatly increases the sample size beyond the target arrived at through power analysis. More is not always better—but, in some instances, the lure of statistical significance seduces researchers into the practice of continually incrementing their sample sizes until statistical significance is reached. When this is done, statistical significance may be reached at an effect size much smaller than that set in the power analysis. Results finally might achieve statistical significance, but the small effect size that has been detected through the power of huge samples might be clinically meaningless.

■ FAMILIES OF COMMON ANALYTIC METHODS

One of the most intimidating aspects of statistics is that there seem to be so many choices. When contemplating the multitude of tests available in inferential statistics, it is easy to feel lost in a sea of analytic methods. Actually, statistical methods can be grouped conceptually so that instead of considering scores of individual statistical tests, the research consumer can think in terms of a few families of statistical methods.

When thinking in terms of families of methods, begin by grasping the simplest statistical tests that represent that family. These simple tests are prototypes of all the other tests, which follow in greater complexity. After you understand the purpose

TABLE 3d FAMILIES OF COMMON ANALYTIC METHODS*

Family I. Differences Between Groups	Family II. Relations Among Variables
If a study was designed to:	
Investigate differences between groups, as in a controlled trial or experiment	Investigate the relations among variables and a health outcome, as in cohort or case-control studies
A typical research question in this family might be:	
Do patients with Stage II breast cancer asssigned to who are randomly adjuvant therapy with tamoxifen live longer than patients who are randomly assigned to adjuvant chemotherapy?	To what extent are diet, exercise, and family history related to the development of coronary artery disease?
Expect to see statistics that:	
Focus on differences in the average responses of the two groups	Focus on the relation of variables to the outcome of interest
Simple examples of such statistics are:	
t tests for differences between two groups	Correlation between two variables tested with z
More complex versions of statistics in this family are:	
F tests for differences between more than two groups	Multiple regression for relations among more than one variable and a health outcome
Analysis of variance (ANOVA): One-way ANOVA, Factorial ANOVA, Multivariate ANOVA, Repeated measures ANOVA	Discriminant analysis
	Canonical correlation
Analysis of covariance (ANCOVA)	

*The concept of families of common analytic methods is the property of T. J. Jordan.

of a particular family of methods, you will see that the more complex statistical methods are merely variations on a rather straightforward theme. Table 3d provides a breakdown of two of the most common families of analytic methods encountered in medical research.

The more complex versions of statistical methods in each family can be understood readily by considering how they build upon each other. Analysis of variance lends itself readily to a working example: Begin with the original research question indicated as an example for Family I.

1. If the question were limited to the differences between patients on tamoxifen versus patients on traditional chemotherapy, a simple t test could be used.

2. Now consider adding a third group: women who have not had any adjuvant therapy. This brings us to a simple F test, or a one-way analysis of variance for three groups.
3. Add a further level of complexity: In addition to three treatment groups, consider Stage I breast cancer separately from Stage II breast cancer. Now we have what is called a factorial analysis of variance, which permits us to see whether the three treatment options have differential effects on the two different stages of disease.
4. Decide that we want to investigate the effects of the three treatments not only on life expectancy but also on quality of life. Using more than one outcome measure in a controlled trial brings us to a multivariate analysis of variance.
5. Because quality of life may change over time, we decide that we want to measure this variable at 6-month intervals for the next 2 years. Since we are measuring quality of life on the same patients several times, we have a repeated measures analysis of variance.
6. Finally, we decide that the age of the woman at time of diagnosis might be a confounding factor in the study. Since we cannot feasibly design a study in which all women are the same age, we decide to use a statistical technique called covariance to take the effects of age out of our findings. This requires an analysis of covariance.

These six steps provide a clue as to how families of analytic methods build in complexity without losing the initial thread or theme of the family. These steps are provided as an illustration. In "real life" they can be combined to give us such methods as multivariate analysis of covariance with repeated measures! Hopefully, you will be able now to translate this into English without being intimidated by the seeming complexity of the method.

The Qualitative–Quantitative Continuum....................................

Medical information, and difficulty understanding medical information, typically involves quantification, i.e., assigning numbers to phenomena and subjecting the resulting data to mathematical analysis. Consequently, the focus of this book, and especially this chapter, is quantitative research. However, the chapter would be incomplete without a brief discussion of the role of qualitative research.

Quantitative research is the legacy of a long history of positivist thinking in the natural sciences about how science should be done. In physics, chemistry, and biology, phenomena are observed and counted. Research is aimed at establishing general laws, and reality is thought to be "objective." From this perspective, the ultimate goal is to find a theory of everything that would sit atop the hierarchy of theories and be comprised only of mathematical equations. Tegmark and Wheeler (2001, p. 75) state: "Crudely speaking, the ratio of equations to words decreases as one moves down the tree, dropping near zero for very applied fields such as medicine and sociology. In contrast, theories near the top are highly mathematical, and physicists are still struggling to comprehend the concepts that are encoded in the mathematics." While some philosophers view medicine as a poor instance of a positivist science, the ways in which medical data are collected, analyzed, and interpreted clearly reflect a positivist legacy (see Foucault, 1994).

Qualitative research is experiencing a wave of enthusiasm in some areas of the social sciences. In reaction to positivist science, qualitative researchers view reality as something that is socially constructed and the aim of research to be understanding. As in quantitative research, there are many types of qualitative research, characterized by different goals and different approaches to the task of making meaning. One thing that is common across most qualitative methods is a reliance on verbal text to obtain the subjective meaning people make of experiences in their lives. An example of qualitative research would be a study designed to further the understanding of how parents of children with serious diseases experience living with this problem. Information could be gathered through open-ended interviews designed to permit the participants maximum breadth in the material they bring to the meaning making task. In some types of qualitative research, texts are "analyzed" to find themes that cut across participants. In other approaches, meta-themes are not sought, and the "story" of each participant speaks for itself. Nearly all qualitative studies enroll only a handful of participants, since there is no need for large numbers in the absence of generalizability as a goal, and when depth of understanding is better served by attending in great detail to the voice of each individual.

In contemporary medicine, there are a multitude of areas in which quantitative research clearly is appropriate. Finding genetic markers linked to cancer, investigating the effect of anti-retroviral therapies on viral load, and measuring the impact of beta blockers on hypertension are examples of areas that require quantification/quantitative research. There are other areas, however, that might better be served by qualitative study. For example, learning about the quality of life of people with chronic diseases, understanding the ways in which children make sense of illness, and describing how families function when a member becomes gravely ill—all could be fertile domains for qualitative study.

Some researchers view qualitative and quantitative research as comprising a continuum, with the possibility that combined qualitative/quantitative studies will yield the richest kinds of results.

Becoming Comfortable with Knowing Less Than Everything

Full textbooks are written on inferential statistics alone, as they are on descriptive statistics, multivariate statistics, research design, and clinical trial methodology. Most of those texts are of the "how to" genre. While learning how to calculate (or, rather, have a computer calculate) an analysis of variance or a multiple regression is extremely helpful—even necessary for active researchers—it is possible to be an excellent consumer of research without knowing everything about every topic mentioned in this chapter.

The old adage says that *a little knowledge is a dangerous thing.* In the area of medical information, it is likely to be more dangerous to have no knowledge at all. Here are some suggestions to help you delve into all aspects of a research report without intimidation:

- Stop worrying about how little you know, and consider how wise it is to recognize the limits of your knowledge.
- Begin to recognize that you are not alone: We live in an age in which everyone feels that they are constantly playing "catch up" with the newest methodologies.
- Come to terms with the fact that it is not possible to be an expert in everything. Good consumers of research who translate what they read responsibly into clinical practice are the most important reason that clinical research is done: so that it can be used to improve the health of populations.
- When you don't understand something, ask for help from someone who does know and is willing to translate the material into English. A related suggestion is to stop equating "I don't understand" with "I'm stupid" or "I'm irresponsible." A desire to learn is neither stupid nor irresponsible.
- Exert the effort it takes to read all parts of research articles. The more you read, the more questions you will have, and the more you will learn.
- Finally, use some common sense. If something seems to be missing from an article, it probably is missing. If analytic methods appear to be overly complex and unintelligible, they probably are: Remember that it is the author's responsibility to make the research report intelligible to a broad audience. And if conclusions do not seem to follow from results, you may have found an unfortunate instance of a rather prevalent problem. Remember that people who serve as reviewers of research

articles often skimp on the same sections that "ordinary" research consumers gloss over!

Suggested References ....

Campbell, D. T., & Stanley, J. C. (1963). *Experimental and quasi-experimental design*. Chicago: Rand McNally. This book provides a comprehensive yet readable discussion of the variations on experimental-type designs. It should be on the personal bookshelves of anyone with an interest in clinical trial methodology. In addition to providing graphic illustrations of every variation on design, it contains excellent discussions of the strengths, weaknesses, and possible threats to validity associated with each. While the focus of the book and the examples it uses are primarily from the social sciences, making the transition to medical studies should not prove difficult.

Daniel, W.W. (1987). *Biostatistics: A foundation for analysis in the health sciences (4th Ed.)*. New York: John Wiley and Sons. There are literally hundreds of statistics books from which to choose when deciding to find a good reference. While this one is dated, it has several strengths: The examples are good teaching examples, i.e., they are readily understood without wading through unnecessary medical jargon. It is organized in a useful and sensible manner. Finally, the ratio of words to numbers is quite high. This means you will be reading explanations, not just formulas.

Newman, I., & Benz, C. R. (1998). *Qualitative–quantitative research methodology*. Carbondale and Edwardsville, IL: Southern Illinois University Press. There are large volumes of edited works on qualitative research that are extremely useful to individuals who are contemplating conducting qualitative studies. For individuals who would like to begin developing an understanding of the differences between the two general approaches as well as the ways in which these approaches might intersect, this short book is a good place to start. The text presents philosophical positions in an easily understandable way, and does a good job covering topics of validity and legitimation.

Riegelman, R.K. (1981). *Studying a study and testing a test*. Boston: Little, Brown and Company. There are two parts of this four-part book that bear directly on the topics discussed in this chapter. The discussions are quite brief, but might provide another way of looking at the same topics—something that can be helpful if you find yourself "stuck" on some of the concepts in research design and statistics.

Citations in Text ....

Bakewin, H. (1945). Pseudodoxia pediatrica. *New England Journal of Medicine, 232(24),* 691-697.

Baltes, P. B., & Nesselroade, J. R. (1979). History and rationale of longitudinal research. In J. R. Nesselroade & P. B. Baltes (Eds.). *Longitudinal research in the study of behavior and development.* New York, Academic Press, Inc.

Corbie-Smith, G. (1999). The continuing legacy of the Tuskeegee syphilis study: Considerations for clinical investigation. *American Journal of Medical Science, 317(1),* 5-8.

Foucault, M. (1994). *The birth of the clinic.* New York: Vintage Books.

Jones, J. (1981). *Bad blood: The Tuskeegee syphilis experiment: A tragedy of race and medicine.* New York: The Free Press.

Konner, M. (1993). *Medicine at the crossroads.* New York: Pantheon Books.

McCarthy C., Sr. (1974). HMO's: Evaluating the pros and cons. Hospital Progress, *55(11),* 50-54.

Steering Committee of the Physicians' Health Study Research Group (1989). Final Report on the aspirin component of the ongoing physicians' health study. *New England Journal of Medicine,* 321: 129-135.

Tegmark, M., & Wheeler, J. A. (2001). 100 years of quantum mysteries. *Scientific American,* February, 68-75.

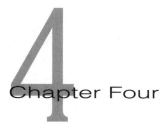

Chapter Four

Generating Diagnoses

Medicine is a science of uncertainty and an art of probability.

Sir William Osler

Introduction

Patients who are experiencing physical complaints ask their physicians what appear to be some very straightforward questions: "What's wrong with me?" " Why do I have pain [or other discomforts]?" "Do I have cancer [or some other disease or condition]?" In medical language, patients present to their physicians with one or more **symptoms,** among which there usually is a **chief complaint.** Symptoms are the patient's subjective experiences that something unusual or abnormal is happening. The most important symptom experienced by the patient, typically the symptom most clearly responsible for initiating a visit to the physician, is the chief complaint. While it is not always easy to separate a chief complaint from an array of symptoms, the task becomes somewhat easier when the chief complaint is thought of as the major reason a patient is seeking medical advice.

When individuals visit their physicians for well-patient check-ups or routine physical examinations, the typical questions may take a somewhat different tone: "Is everything alright?" "Am I in good shape [healthy]?" "How is my heart [or some other organ]?" In these cases, the focus is not identification of a chief complaint or making a diagnosis, but rather obtaining evidence to assure that everything is alright. Often, on a routine physical examination (not an exam prompted by symptoms), diseases are found **incidentally,** that is, without the specific intention to make a diagnosis. For example, hypertension may be diagnosed during a routine physical examination in the absence of patient complaints, since hypertension frequently is asymptomatic.

Medical decisions typically take a "go/no-go" form. This means that while probabilities are taken into consideration when making a diagnostic (or therapeutic) choice, the choice itself amounts to doing something versus doing nothing, or taking one course of action instead of another: e.g., order an MRI or watch and wait, perform a fine needle biopsy or an open excisional biopsy, elect empiric therapy to help confirm a diagnosis or continue diagnostic testing.

Health care providers may answer patients' health questions with "yes" or "no" answers, even when the questions might be extremely difficult, complex, and based on multiple probabilities. The most fundamental reason for these dichotomous responses is the go/no-go nature of medical action. Even deciding to do nothing is a course of action that comprises one half of a dichotomy, e.g., a decision must be made to begin treatment now or to withhold it until further tests are performed. Withholding treatment is a decision not to treat, just as treating a disease or performing a diagnostic test is deciding on a course of action.

In spite of the important role of probabilities in medical reasoning, patients often have learned to expect dichotomous, go/no-go answers from their physicians. In addition to the go/no-go nature of medical action, numerous social factors contribute to the dichotomous kind of dialogue that occurs between patient and physician. Some patients more readily trust a physician who does not qualify or "hedge" the answers, a physician who avoids talking in terms of probabilities. This may be due in part to a lack of training of the lay public about the probabilistic nature of medicine and the desire to view medicine as a science of certainty. Other patients may prefer the physician to assume an authoritarian rather than a collaborative role and simply tell them what to do. And physicians frequently experience psychological discomfort with the degree of uncertainty that underlies many medical decisions. (See Chapter 2, The Nature of Medical Reasoning and the Limits of Medical Information.)

Not all patients' medical problems pose diagnostic challenges. A 45-year-old patient rushed to the nearest emergency room because he has received a gunshot wound to his shoulder typically does not pose an intellectually challenging diagnostic dilemma. Diagnosis: Traumatic injury to left clavicle area pursuant to gunshot. Most likely, the critical issues will involve life-saving treatment procedures, including cessation of blood loss, treatment of shock responses, and assessment and repair of damage to critical organs.

Now consider the following scenario: The same (gunshot) patient, having recovered with no disabling mechanical or organic difficulties, returns to his personal physician 5 years later complaining of pain in his left arm. On the surface, his question appears quite simple: "Has my arm begun to hurt because of that gunshot wound to my shoulder 5 years ago?" For the physician, an answer is likely to be more difficult than a simple, "yes, of course." Instead, the physician considers a number of possibilities, correlated with varying degrees of severity and leading to dramatically different diagnostic and treatment options. A few of the diagnostic options might include: osteoarthritis in the shoulder joint, a completely new injury such as a strain or sprain, and signs of an imminent heart attack given the gender and age of the patient.

Now the physician is confronted with a diagnostic problem. It seems quite likely that a traumatic gunshot injury to bone could very well result in arthritic changes over a 5-year period. On the other hand, patients are certainly "entitled" to more than one disease process. Perhaps there is a new injury occurring in addition to arthritis, something that might result in a sensation of muscle soreness or pain. On the other hand, this physical complaint could signal a medical emergency, i.e., a serious cardiovascular event.

As the patient waits for his "yes or no" answer, the physician considers that more information is necessary, and the process of making a diagnosis begins.

Narrowing the Possibilities and Generating a Differential Diagnosis ....

■ USING VERBAL REPORTS TO NARROW POSSIBILITIES

> Listen carefully to your patients. They will tell you the diagnosis.
>
> Sir William Osler

Often, patients as well as health care providers think of medical tests as procedures that require the use of medical equipment, ranging from noninvasive techniques such as applying a stethoscope to hear heart sounds, to slightly invasive laboratory tests such as obtaining blood samples by venipuncture, to highly invasive tests such as performing excisional biopsies usually with local or general anesthesia (e.g., biopsy of breast or any internal organ, bone marrow biopsy, skin biopsy).

However, many other kinds of information can comprise medical tests, particularly when a medical test is thought of as any vehicle that can help in narrowing down the number of a patient's possible diagnoses. A good patient history, obtained simply through discussion, serves as an important medical "test." A good history covers the patient's own illness and wellness "biography" as well as information about relatives and close contacts. Knowing about biological relatives can provide useful information for assessing increased risk for certain diseases, such as heart disease, hypertension, arthritis, and particular types of cancer. Information about close contacts, while not a source of clues about inherited or genetic predispositions, can provide useful knowledge about the possibilities of infectious contacts and increased risks for such diseases as tuberculosis and HIV.

In a health history, time frames can also play an important role: If a 45-year-old patient reports that her mother experienced early menopause (in her 40s), there is an increased likelihood that the patient's complaints of severe headaches, sweats, dizziness, nervousness, and one missed menstrual period in the absence of pregnancy might be harbingers of early menopause for her. If a patient's father had his first heart attack at age 50, the pains the patient is describing in his chest may, nevertheless, be transient sore muscles related to that refrigerator he unloaded from a truck the other day, but also could have cardiac causes. On the other hand, since he was furious that he got stuck unloading that monster himself, his chest pains also might be related to psychological causes (which may, in turn, help trigger cardiac problems as well as muscle injury.) If a patient's biological mother developed invasive breast cancer at age 35, the patient might very well consider beginning mammographic screening earlier in her life than is recommended for the general population, and might consider having mammograms done more frequently than what is recommended for women without familial risks. And if no one can make sense of why a patient ended up in the hospital with an excruciating pain in his back, it might be because he failed to tell his physicians about that car accident 25 years ago that sent him to physical therapy for a suspected lumbar disk problem in the days when diagnostic imaging with MRI was unavailable.

A thorough medical history also will require as much information as the patient can provide about present and past health-related behavior patterns. These might include consumption of prescription and nonprescription medications, street drugs, and alcohol. Family information on these topics can also be useful. The medical history will probably cover sexual preferences and behaviors, questions that do not always elicit honest answers from the patient because they can create discomfort and a sense that the physician is needlessly "prying."

One of the crucial roles of a health history, including information about family and close contacts, is that the information can be used to estimate a particular patient's risk or likelihood of having or getting a particular disease. Consider, for example, that the general risk (the risk estimate for the general population of women in the United States) of developing breast cancer during their lifetimes is approximately 1 in 8, or about 12%. The presence of breast cancer in a first-degree relative (mother, sister, daughter) raises that risk substantially. If the patient is found to carry mutations of a known breast cancer gene, her likelihood of developing breast cancer during her lifetime might be estimiated at virtually 100%; and she is more likely to develop breast cancer earlier in her life than women without the presently identifiable genetic mutations. In this example, a health history establishing breast cancer in a first-degree relative can provide direction for an optimal screening regimen, i.e., an individual recommendation about the use of *medical tests.*

Since patient responses to medical history questions can provide important diagnostic information, it is often useful to know something about how the medical history was taken: Was enough time given to obtain full information? Or was the patient rushed through the history because the physician's schedule was very tight? Was the patient encouraged to engage in a discourse with the physician, or did he or she feel intimidated and "cut off" by the physician's lack of eye-contact as she typed the history into the computer instead of focusing on the patient? Was the history taken in private? Or was it done in the presence of another family member, or in an open cubicle instead of a closed office? Was confidentiality of sensitive information assured?

To a great extent, a patient's medical history constitutes **self-report data.** In order for self-report data to be accurate, the patient must be both willing and able to answer the questions that are posed. For example, if a patient who has been treated by several physicians for a multitude of medical problems including hypertension, arthritis, menopausal symptoms, and chronic pain, is asked to report which medications at which dosages she has taken during the past 10 years, she simply may be unable to provide an accurate report because the amount of information is impossible to recall. Consider, on the other hand, a 19-year-old patient who is brought into an emergency room by his mother because he has what appears to be pneumonia, and has been losing weight for no clear reason during the past several months. With mom standing next to the stretcher in the ER, a physician takes a quick history, covering sexual habits and drug use in detail because the patient may have HIV disease. The patient denies sexual activity of any kind, since he is unwilling to report his homosexual orientation in the presence of his mother. What might have been crucial information in diagnosing and treating this patient has been lost, and clinching a diagnosis will be delayed, because the "test" of medical history is inaccurate. In acute care situations, as in an emergency room, it may be impossible to obtain an adequate history. Information obtained under less than optimal conditions must be regarded as circumspect.

■USING PREVALENCE AS A DIAGNOSTIC TEST

The term **prevalence** refers to the amount of disease that is thought to exist in a particular population. It takes into account individuals who have a particular medical condition at a given moment in time, meaning that it takes into consideration "old" cases that were diagnosed some time in the past in patients who are still alive as well as "new" cases that have been diagnosed within the year.

Prevalence differs from **incidence,** a term that refers only to new cases of a disease. When reports of increases or decreases in such diseases as tuberculosis and HIV infection are reported, it is usually incidence that is of greatest concern. When reports of breast cancer risk inform women in the United States that they have a 1 in 8 risk of developing breast cancer during their lifetimes, prevalence of breast cancer has been used to derive this estimate. Yearly, or incident, cases of breast cancer represent fewer than 1 of every 8 U.S. women. If 1 in 8 were incidence rather than prevalence, this would mean that 8 years from now, every woman in the United States would have breast cancer.

Prevalence can serve as a kind of diagnostic test because it helps to set the base line risk for a patient at a given site. What this means is that a patient who comes to an emergency room in an urban center in the northeastern United States with complaints of fever, swollen lymph glands, weight loss without dieting, and a history of intravenous drug use would have a relatively high risk of being infected with HIV because HIV infection is prevalent among intravenous drug users in urban centers in the northeastern United States. Here the "background" prevalence helps in formulating diagnostic hypotheses.

Similarly, if a suburban patient in the midwestern United States with no history of intravenous drug use or risky sexual behavior complained of fever and swollen glands, the prevalence of HIV in her sub-population would be sufficiently low to convince health care workers to pursue other diagnostic hypotheses, such as mononucleosis rather than HIV infection.

Information about the prevalence of a disease in a given population may be used to provide general guidance about how to narrow a diagnosis. However, making the jump from population figures to diagnosis of an individual case can be very problematic because differences among individuals within a population can be vast (See Chapter 5 on Assessing the Health of Populations). Similarly, incidence figures can be helpful in alerting the health care community to increases or decreases in the types of disease they are likely to encounter in their patients. Like prevalence, however, incidence provides only very general guidance on what to expect. The midwestern patient might have contracted HIV disease through risky sexual contacts that she did not report, and the urban intravenous drug user may be infected with tuberculosis and may be HIV-seronegative.

■THE WHY'S AND HOW'S OF NARROWING DIAGNOSTIC OPTIONS

In an example used above, a woman aged 45 complained to her physician of severe headaches, sweats, dizziness, and nervousness. She also reported that her mother experienced menopause during her 40s. In this case, it appears rather likely that the patient is experiencing the onset of menopause. Some blood work to assess hormone levels could be a straightforward way to help determine her status. Other "easy" diagnostic modalities might consist of a watch-and-wait approach to see whether she misses more than the one menstrual period already reported. Given the family history plus rather clear symptoms, some physicians would put this patient on a trial of hormone replacement therapy consisting of both estrogen and progesterone. If she responded positively to hormone replacement therapy, i.e., her symptoms were alleviated, this empiric therapy could be taken as evidence that the diagnosis of early menopause was correct. (On the other hand, as is typical in contemporary medicine, there are arguments against—as well as for—hormone replacement therapy, including possible increased risks for some kinds of cancer. These arguments might dissuade the patient and/or the physician from using empiric therapy.)

Since many of this patient's symptoms, including her chief complaint of headache, are consistent with a diagnosis of menopause, many physicians would take no further diagnostic/therapeutic steps than those mentioned above. This approach is consistent with a popular adage in clinical medicine, which goes something like this: When you hear hoofbeats, look for horses before you look for zebras. In other words, consider a diagnosis that is common and likely before an uncommon, unlikely one. What is considered common versus uncommon relates closely to the "background" risk rates expressed in estimates of disease incidence and prevalence.

There is wisdom in this kind of diagnostic reasoning. It limits the discomfort, cost, risk, and inconvenience that may very well be unnecessary in making a correct diagnosis. While cost containment has become a critical issue in American medicine, remember that some diagnostic tests are avoided not only because of cost but also because the tests themselves can be risky and even life threatening.

In the case of the woman with headache, sweats, dizziness, and nervousness, the likelihood that she will undergo menopause during a normal life expectancy is 100%. The likelihood that she is beginning menopause now, and that early menopause is the correct diagnosis, is quite high given her family history. An estimate that early menopause is the cause of her symptoms might be as high as 90+%.

On the other hand, sometimes hoofbeats truly mean zebras! This patient's symptoms, particularly her severe headaches, are also consistent with a diagnosis of meningioma, a rather rare brain tumor. The likelihood that she has a meningioma is somewhat less than .3%. In other words, her symptoms are nonspecific, meaning that they can occur in more than one disease, including the natural life event of menopause as well as meningioma, which is unusual but can be life threatening if untreated. Furthermore, some meningiomas contain estrogen and progesterone receptors, making the use of hormone replacement therapy dangerous if not life threatening. Consequently, if a diagnosis of early menopause were made, and the patient were placed on hormone replacement therapy, it is possible that a meningioma would tumorize further or faster due to increased hormones, making surgical removal of the tumor and resultant cure more difficult if not impossible to achieve.

Which diagnostic modalities would be necessary in order to determine if this patient has a meningioma instead of or along with early menopause? The diagnostic work-up could include: CT (computed tomography), MRI (magnetic resonance imaging), MRI enhanced with a contrast medium (gadolinium-DTPA), and MRA (magnetic resonance angiography). These tests, particularly the last two, have invasive components and can pose risks to the patient.

At this point, the physician has a strong hypothesis, also called a **working diagnosis**, which is that the patient's symptoms are symptoms of early menopause. This working diagnosis has been made on the basis of several factors:

1. The patient's symptoms are consistent with menopause.
2. While age 45 is somewhat early for menopause, it is not extremely early or unusual, since most women in the

United States begin menopause at approximately age
50.

3. Her biological mother experienced menopause during
her 40s.

4. The patient has not complained of any additional symptoms that would suggest an increased likelihood of brain
tumor, such as disturbance in visual field or vomiting.
(However, the physician recognizes that these latter
symptoms might not occur in early stages of neurological brain disease.)

In this process, the physician has narrowed the hypothesis
to menopause. In other words, the physician has heard hoofbeats and has looked for horses instead of zebras. Next, this
working diagnosis or hypothesis must be challenged by other
possibilities.

■DIFFERENTIAL DIAGNOSIS AND THE POSSIBLE SEARCH FOR ZEBRAS

In a sense, developing a differential diagnosis is like playing
"devil's advocate" with one's own diagnostic reasoning. Taking
a different perspective, the physician asks which other diseases
(besides the one that is hypothesized as a working diagnosis)
might be possible. In the above example of the woman who is
hypothesized to be undergoing menopause, a competing "explanation" would be a neurological disease (a brain tumor, such
as the one mentioned, is a possible candidate).

However, generating a differential diagnosis is not limited
to a working (hypothesized) diagnosis versus one other possibility. Instead, the task of the diagnostician is to consider all
possible and reasonable alternate diseases that might explain
the patient's complaints.

How does one decide which alternatives are possible and
reasonable? Or, virtually impossible and unreasonable? Here
are a few guidelines that are used in making the differential diagnosis appropriately inclusive without containing unnecessary

possibilities that would require further (probably unnecessary) work-ups.

1. Avoid dengue fever, cholera, malaria, and other such diseases that are endemic only in particular parts of the world, unless a patient has traveled in endemic areas or has emigrated from such an area.

2. Conversely, be certain to obtain information regarding the patient's travels and contacts. If a patient has traveled in areas in which malaria is endemic, even if she has taken antimalarial therapy, her fever and sweats may be symptoms of a resistant strain of the disease.

3. Be familiar with gender, age, life-style, and race-associated propensities for particular diseases. For example, Kaposi's sarcoma in an elderly Jewish man may simply be Kaposi's sarcoma, while Kaposi's sarcoma in a 25-year-old gay male may signal the presence of HIV disease.

4. Avoid searching for rare disease alternatives unless there is a reason. For example, primary hemochromatosis is a relatively rare genetic error of metabolism present in approximately 3 to 8 per 1000 individuals. It is a disease that results in increased absorption of iron. Since iron deficiencies are far more common than iron overload, and iron deficiencies are more common in women than in men, one would probably not include hemochromatosis in a differential diagnosis in a young woman complaining of fatigue unless her family history revealed the presence of this genetically determined error.

5. Even when a disease alternative is quite unlikely, it should be considered for inclusion in the differential diagnosis when missing the disease could result in irreversible, serious consequences. A 30-year-old woman who exercises regularly, appears in excellent health, and has no history of cardiovascular disease in self or family, but suddenly complains of severe chest pain accompanied by nausea

should be worked up for a heart attack. While this patient appears an unlikely candidate for heart attack, the consequence of failing to consider heart attack in the differential diagnosis could be mortality.

6. Be thoughtful about the cases you, the health care provider, have seen most recently or those that have impressed you in a way that "remains with you" throughout your practice. Even the best health care professionals can be unduly influenced by personal experience and anecdote, as opposed to more accurate probabilistic reasoning and statistical inference. For example, a physician who had seen an 11-year-old child die from what was later found to be the relatively rare long QT syndrome (a genetic abnormality of the heart's electrical system), might be more likely to overdiagnose this syndrome in other youngsters who have fainted (one manifestation of long QT syndrome).

Testing to Finalize a Diagnosis

■ORDERING MEDICAL TESTS

At some point in the diagnostic process, the physician will have arrived at a working diagnosis (or hypothesis) plus a differential (alternative explanations). The amount of effort it takes to arrive at this point, as well as the number and complexity of the procedures that will be necessary to establish a final diagnosis, depend on a number of factors including:

1. How difficult it is to diagnose the particular disease
2. The likelihood that a disease is "presenting" itself in an atypical way
3. The presence of coexisting medical problems
4. The tests and technology available to assist in arriving at an accurate diagnosis

Earlier in this chapter, the roles of symptoms and chief complaints were discussed in the context of developing a differential diagnosis. To understand better the role of medical testing, it is essential to include the additional concepts of signs and causes.

Recall that symptoms are defined as a patient's sense that something is wrong, painful, uncomfortable, or abnormal/unusual in some way. The key here is that symptoms typically refer to the patient's perceptions and, while extremely important are, nevertheless, subjective. In addition to this subjective information, the physician is also likely to seek objective sources of information, called **signs.** In contrast to symptoms of a disease, signs of a disease are objective sources of information uncovered by the physician during a physical exam and/or during the process of follow-up testing. This follow-up testing typically is referred to as "working a patient up" or a "work up" for a disease. Bear in mind that sometimes the distinction between signs and symptoms may be a difficult one: *Stedman's Medical Dictionary* states that a sign is "an objective symptom of a disease, in contrast to a symptom, which is a subjective sign of a disease."

Frequently, patients are puzzled about why the physician orders "additional" medical tests after a diagnosis is made. Consider, for example, a 50-year-old man who presents to his physician with a chief complaint of sensations of pressure in his head. During the physical examination, the physician performs the noninvasive medical test for hypertension and discovers that the patient does, in fact, have elevated systolic and diastolic blood pressures, making a diagnosis of hypertension consistent with his symptom. At this point, there is "agreement" between the patient's subjective complaint and the objective sign of hypertension obtained through a medical test. Now, the patient expects to receive a prescription for antihypertensive medication.

However, the patient's medical history reveals no hypertension in any family members. Since hypertension is often familial, and since hypertension usually is asymptomatic, the physician is uncomfortable treating this patient's hypertension with traditional medical therapy in the absence of additional tests. To the patient's dismay, the physician orders a battery of further tests, perhaps including a complete blood count, a urinalysis, blood levels of creatinine, potassium, uric acid, etc., and an ECG (electrocardiogram) as starters! Why? In the absence of familial hypertension and in the presence of a troubling symptom, it is possible that this patient's hypertension is caused by something other than the typical hemodynamic and pathophysiologic derangements that result in what is called primary or essential hypertension, the kind of hypertension best treated with antihypertensive drugs. This patient may have secondary hypertension, that is, hypertension caused by other factors such as occlusion of the renal (kidney) arteries, which may be corrected through surgical intervention, or even malignant hypertension, which untreated typically results in mortality within 1 year. What the physician has done is generate a differential diagnosis by considering the patient's chief complaint (symptom), information obtained in the medical history, and the sign of hypertension derived from a single medical test.

Sometimes identifying a cause can result in a more refined diagnosis, for example, altering a patient's diagnosis from hypertension to renovascular hypertension. In other instances, identifying a cause may not alter or refine the diagnosis. In either event, identifying the cause of a disease, which is not always the same thing as making a diagnosis, plays an essential role in treatment decisions. Diagnosis alone is giving a name or attaching a label to the patient's condition. Sometimes it is not possible to go further: For example, the true causes of primary or essential hypertension are poorly understood, and medical therapy is initiated despite this lack of precise knowledge. In other instances, giving a name or label to a disease may not provide sufficient direction for treatment, which is the major role of diagnosis. In order to treat a disease optimally, it is essential to know either the underlying cause of the disease or that the underlying cause is simply unknowable given the present state of medical research but that some forms of treatment may be available. When the underlying cause can be removed, the most successful treatment is likely to be achieved.

To summarize what has been discussed in this section, diagnostic tests serve as relatively objective indicators of the presence (or absence) of disease. The physician runs routine tests, such as blood pressure assessments, and may order special tests, such as an ECG, to help "clinch" a working diagnosis or to explore the possibilities suggested by a differential diagnosis.

■**USING AND INTERPRETING MEDICAL TESTS—BASIC CONCEPTS AND TEST CHARACTERISTICS**

Medical tests have two fundamental purposes: to rule in and to rule out diseases. For example, it is recommended that middle-aged women have base-line mammograms, usually with annual follow-up mammograms, to rule in the possibility of breast cancer. Abnormal results on mammograms will occur in many women; only a fraction of these women with abnormal tests will have breast cancer. However, women with abnormal or "suspicious" mammograms will be sent for breast biopsies to rule out the possibility of breast cancer.

At first, this kind of medical reasoning may seem counter-intuitive. Why try to rule-in diseases and then try to rule them out? Here, a translation of medical terms into everyday language can be helpful. By ruling in a disease, diagnosticians try to cast as wide a net as possible in order to be sure that no one who might have a particular disease is missed (especially a disease like breast cancer, which is very serious but also potentially curable in early stages). The important first step is to "catch" as many people as possible who could have the disease—and since breast cancer is a common disease among women, mammograms are recommended for all women beginning in middle-age. It is well known that mammograms will "catch" many healthy women in the net of "possible cancers." (In fact, mammography has been criticized for casting too wide a net and resulting in too many ruling-in procedures, i.e., biopsies for many women who do not have cancer.)

When a wide net is cast to rule in possible disease, the next phase must be to rule out disease in individuals who are healthy, so that only those individuals who require treatment will be treated. In the breast cancer example, women with abnormal mammograms are sent for breast biopsies to obtain tissue samples of the areas that appear suspicious. These biopsies may be performed through the insertion of a biopsy needle into an identified area, or as "open-biopsies," which are surgical procedures. The tissue samples obtained through biopsy will be examined microscopically to see if cancer cells are present. If cancer cells are seen, then the test used to rule out breast cancer has, in fact, established a clear diagnosis of breast cancer!

The language of ruling in and ruling out diseases can be misleading. It is helpful to focus on the basic principles at issue rather than the medical jargon: Very rarely are medical tests good at both identifying all individuals who might have a disease, as well as zeroing in on those who actually have the disease. Consequently, diagnostic testing often proceeds in steps or stages, going from tests that cast a wide net and are called **sensitive,** to tests that are much more stringent in omitting healthy individuals and are called **specific.**

The more sensitive a medical test, the more likely it will produce errors of inclusion, that is, including people as possibly having a disease when they are actually healthy. When a test result is positive, suggesting that someone has a disease, but the person does not actually have the disease, the result is called a false positive. When a false positive occurs, a healthy person may be subjected unnecessarily to further, invasive testing or even to treatment for a disease he or she does not have.

The more specific a medical test, the more likely it is to produce errors of exclusion, that is indicating that people are healthy when they actually have the disease in question. When a test result is negative, suggesting that no disease is present, but the person really does have the disease in question, the result is called a false negative. When a false negative occurs, a diagnosis is missed, usually resulting in failure to provide the patient with appropriate and timely treatment for the disease.

The sensitivity and specificity of diagnostic tests, as well as false-positive and false-negative results, are quantifiable; and they can be used in calculations to determine the likelihood that someone does or does not have a disease. (See section on Probabilities and Calculations below.) False positives and false negatives are errors in diagnosis, and they are minimized by selecting appropriate medical tests.

Medical tests used to rule in diseases typically—but not always—differ from tests used to rule out diseases in a number of important ways, which are summarized in Table 4a.

If issues of cost, risk, and invasiveness are set aside for a moment, the most useful of all tests are those that most clearly and exactly establish the presence of a disease, as in **pathognomonic findings.** An example of a pathognomonic finding is seeing cancer cells present in a tissue biopsy. If cancer cells are present, cancer exists.

There is an additional point that must be kept in mind when considering the steps involved in using medical tests to help finalize a diagnosis: Some diseases are identified by **diagnoses of exclusion.** This means that there are no tests presently in existence that can help to clinch a final diagnosis. Said another way, there are no tests specific for the disease. An example of this kind of situation occurs when a patient complains of very general problems, including fatigue, lethargy, and lack of energy to perform daily tasks. One possibility is that the patient has chronic fatigue syndrome. There are no tests specifically for chronic fatigue syndrome. Instead, the diagnostician can only rule out other diseases included in the differential diagno-

TABLE 4a SUMMARY OF DIFFERENCES BETWEEN SENSITIVE AND SPECIFIC TESTS

Tests for Ruling in Disease	Tests for Ruling Out Disease
Are more sensitive	Are more specific
Cast a wide net	Narrow the net
Produce false positives	Produce false negatives
Are less invasive	Are more invasive
Are less risky	Are more risky
Cost less	Cost more

sis, perhaps depression, iron-deficiency anemia, Lyme disease, and a variety of other infectious processes. If the results of a number of relevant medical tests show normal results, e.g., normal hematocrit levels in the blood indicating the absence of iron-deficiency anemia, a diagnosis of chronic fatigue syndrome may be made because nothing else has been found to account for the patient's symptoms. Diagnoses of exclusion are difficult to make because they often involve many tests; and they are difficult to "trust" because they have not be made directly, such as by visualization of abnormal cells. Consequently, diagnoses of exclusion are often held with a substantial degree of uncertainty.

■USING AND INTERPRETING MEDICAL TESTS—PROBABILITIES AND CALCULATIONS

This chapter began with a discussion of the fact that medical action tends to fit a go/no-go form, which winds up being dichotomous in spite of the complex probabilities that may be involved. Treatment for a disease is either initiated or withheld. The patient expects a "yes" or "no" answer to the question of whether he or she has a particular disease. Sometimes the process of diagnosis is easy; very often it is difficult, requiring more than one stage of information gathering and testing. To arrive at the point of dichotomous action (to treat or not to treat), often requires mathematical calculations to arrive at a best guess regarding the patient's health status.

Sensitivity and specificity, the terms discussed above, are called "test characteristics," and are usually calculated on large groups of people who are already known either to have or not have a given disease. Results of these large-sample studies can be used to assist in making diagnoses for individual patients or other groups of patients.

Studies have shown, for example, that the presence of abnormal amounts of blood in the stool can serve as an indicator of colorectal cancer, so tests for occult blood in the stool can be used to cast a wide net to rule in people who might have the disease and should be worked up further. (Such studies are also used to determine what constitutes "normal" versus what constitutes "abnormal" amounts of blood. Issues of what is normal or abnormal are discussed in greater detail in chapter 5 on Assessing the Health of Populations.) While "catching" 80% of people with colorectal cancer through the presence of blood in the stool might not be as broad a net as one would ideally like, there are factors that argue in favor of this less-than-perfect test: It is easy, inexpensive, noninvasive, and convenient for patients who collect the samples at home by themselves.

Approximately 80% of individuals who have colorectal cancer have higher than normal amounts of blood in samples of their stool. What does this mean in the language of test characteristics? Testing for what is called occult blood in the stool successfully "catches" 80% of individuals with colorectal cancer. This means that the test is 80% **sensitive.** So, if there are 10 people with colorectal cancer, testing for occult blood in the stool will correctly identify or "catch" 8 of them, as illustrated in Figure 4a.

Sensitivity of a test may also be called its **true positive rate** because it is a ratio of the people who are identified correctly by the test ("true positive" people) to the total number of people

Cancer caught: **Cancer missed:**

Calculating *sensitivity* from the above can be represented graphically as

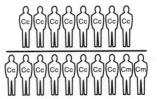   = $\dfrac{8}{10}$ =   80%

Figure 4a Detecting colorectal cancer through occult blood.

who have the disease, including those missed by the test ("true positive" people plus the test's errors, called "false negative" people).

Translating this to the level of the individual patient, it is 80% likely that a patient with colorectal cancer will have a positive test result, indicating possible cancer.

However, there are many other causes for abnormal levels of blood in the stool besides colorectal cancer: These include such factors as having gastritis or bleeding gums. Consequently, the test is likely to make a number of errors, giving positive results in many people who do not have colorectal cancer. This error rate may be as high as 40%. This point is illustrated in Figure 4b in a group of 10 healthy people (without colorectal cancer).

The specificity of this test is 60%. It represents the ratio of people who are identified by the test as not having the disease ("true negative" people) to the total number of people who do not have the disease ("true negative" people plus the test's errors—people who are mistakenly identified as having the disease, the "false positive" people.)

From these illustrations, it is possible to see that testing for blood in the stool can be used as an initial test to rule in the

Healthy people correctly diagnosed as negative:

Healthy people misdiagnosed as positive:

This illustration can assist in calculating the *specificity* of the test:

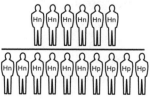 = $\dfrac{6}{10}$ = 60%

Figure 4b Missing a diagnosis of colorectal cancer in healthy people.

possibility of colorectal cancer (although it is not perfect because it will miss 20% of people with the disease.) If this test is used to rule in patients, it will make quite a number of false-positive errors. That is, it will identify a large proportion of people as having colorectal cancer who do not have the disease. As discussed in the previous section, further testing would be needed to rule out colorectal cancer (and to "clinch" or finalize the diagnosis in people who really do have the disease). The further tests used in the diagnostic work up of colorectal cancer are more invasive and include direct visualization of the colon and rectum through colonoscopy.

Sensitivity and specificity are undoubtedly important concepts in the process of ruling in and ruling out disease. However, it is crucial to remember that sensitivity is calculated on individuals already known to have a disease. It tells you how good a test is in identifying disease in a group of diseased individuals. Similarly, specificity is calculated on individuals already known to be disease-free (or healthy). Specificity tells you how good a test is in identifying individuals who do not have a disease in a group of disease-free people.

In the real world, in many clinical situations, it is important to know more than the sensitivity and specificity of a test. Remember, in making a diagnosis, the physician does not know in advance whether a disease is present or absent—the point of ordering a test is to help determine presence or absence of disease. Hopefully, this point will make clear the need for two additional concepts: positive predictive value and negative predictive value.

Predictive values are derived, in part, from the sensitivities and specificities of medical tests. In other words, sensitivities and specificities are not cast aside, but rather provide information that is integrated into the further calculations of predictive values. **Predictive values** differ from sensitivities and specificities in that they are designed to estimate the likelihood that a disease is present or absent when the person being tested is not from a group already known to have a disease or to be disease-free.

In the illustrations used to calculate sensitivity and specificity, symbols were used to indicate people who had cancer and people who were healthy/without cancer. When a cancer was caught, it was represented as Cc; when it was missed as Cm. When a healthy individual was correctly diagnosed as negative for the disease, the finding was represented as Hn; when the diagnosis was incorrectly positive, it was indicated as Hp.

Now, consider that in the real world, patients do not come into physicians' offices with little C's, H's, c's, m's, n's, and p's to indicate their health status and/or accuracy of test findings. While it is true that some diseases present signs that are directly observable by the physician (e.g., advanced Hansen's disease, also called leprosy), medical tests are most useful in the vast majority of diseases that are not so clearly discernible.

Carrying further the example of colorectal cancer (see Figure 4c), assume that 100 patients visit a particular clinic. Think of them as X's, a symbol frequently used in mathematics to designate "unknowns." However, for ease of interpretation, this illustration will use numbers rather than X's. Remember that the critical task is to sort them into groups indicating their health status.

In this example, all 100 patients are over age 60, have a strong family history of colorectal cancer, and show evidence of unexplained blood loss in their blood counts. Thus, it makes sense to suspect and to test for colorectal cancer. For this example, let us assume that these patients are at especially high risk for colorectal cancer, with a likelihood of 50% that cancer is present even before a work up for the disease is begun. The task is to use medical tests to sort these "unknowns" into those who have colorectal cancer and those who do not. Remember, from above, that our first test for colorectal cancer, the test for blood in the stool, is 80% sensitive and 60% specific.

Now the sorting process is performed, given the use of a test for abnormal levels of blood in the stool; and predictive values can be derived. If a patient, previously an unknown X, had a positive result on the medical test, his or her likelihood of having colorectal cancer is Cc divided by Cc plus Hp (everyone

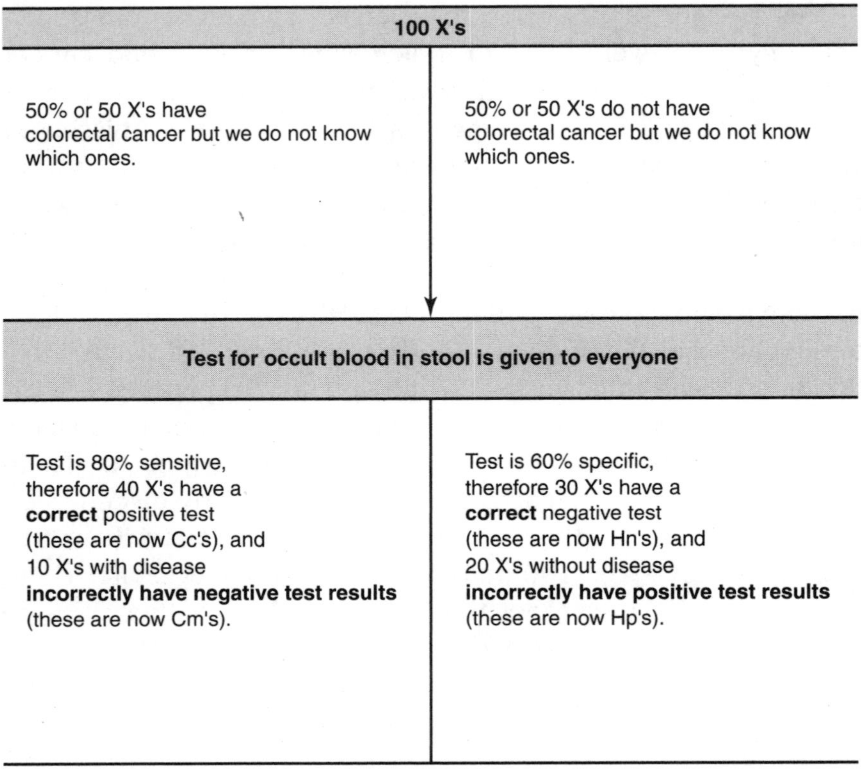

100 X's	
50% or 50 X's have colorectal cancer but we do not know which ones.	50% or 50 X's do not have colorectal cancer but we do not know which ones.

Test for occult blood in stool is given to everyone	
Test is 80% sensitive, therefore 40 X's have a **correct** positive test (these are now Cc's), and 10 X's with disease **incorrectly have negative test results** (these are now Cm's).	Test is 60% specific, therefore 30 X's have a **correct** negative test (these are now Hn's), and 20 X's without disease **incorrectly have positive test results** (these are now Hp's).

Figure 4c Predicting presence and absence of colorectal cancer when health status is unknown.

with a positive test, whether correct or incorrect.) Numerically, this is 40 divided by 40 plus 20, which gives a positive predictive value of 67%. This means that the estimate for an unknown X's likelihood of having colorectal cancer has risen from 50% to 67% given a positive test result.

The same reasoning applies to negative test results. If a patient, previously an unclassified X, had a negative result on the medical test, his or her likelihood of being cancer-free is Hn divided by Hn plus Cm (everyone who had a negative test result, whether correct or incorrect). Numerically, this is 30 divided by

30 plus 10, which gives a negative predictive value of 75%. This means that the estimate for an unknown X's likelihood of not having cancer has risen from 50% to 75%.

Predictive values are only estimates, and they depend to a great extent on the test characteristics of sensitivity and specificity as well as on the risk of the disease patients are assumed to carry before a medical test is performed. (Chapter 5 on Assessing the Health of Populations provides additional information on these risk estimates and covers further the concepts of incidence and prevalence.) However, these estimates can be extremely helpful in medical decisions about whether to continue with further diagnostic testing or whether to stop testing because more tests are unlikely to yield better predictions.

What is particularly interesting, and perhaps troubling, about the crucial concepts of positive and negative predictive values is the fact that they are estimated probabilities. From these estimates, the physician must, once again, arrive at go/no-go decisions.

■RELIABILITY OF DIAGNOSTIC TESTS

Broadly speaking, **reliability** refers to the extent to which the health care provider can be confident that information obtained from a diagnostic test is "robust," unlikely to change from time to time depending on the mood of the patient, the biases of the person reading the X-ray film, the setting in which a measurement was taken, or any other irrelevant factors that might impact on the test results.

Reliability of Patient Reports

In the social sciences, when much that is measured consists of hypothetical constructs (such as motivation, self-concept, anxiety), a great deal of attention is focused on developing measurement tools that will elicit the same responses regardless of who is administering them, where they are being done, whether the patient is tired or hungry, or any number of other extraneous factors.

To determine the reliability of measurements used in the social sciences, they often are administered more than once, and the responses are correlated with each other to see the extent of "match" between them. The higher the correlation, the more reliable the instrument because responses to it have not been affected by extraneous factors.

In the practice of medicine, some of the same kinds of instruments may be used to obtain self-reports of depression, anxiety, psychotic features, pain perceptions, etc.

Inter- and Intra-Rater Reliability

It is not unusual for a radiologist to read the same X-ray differently if he or she has the opportunity to see it again after a period of time has passed. Similarly, a second radiologist may read the X-ray differently from the first radiologist, even if they are equivalently trained and reading it on the same day.

Because there is a great deal of uncertainty in medicine, there is room for different opinions among health care providers, just as there is room for a given professional to differ from him/herself if given the opportunity to review a diagnostic test more than once.

Importance of the Setting

The same diagnostic test might yield substantially different results when administered under different conditions. A classic example is hypertension. Most health care providers realize that simply the idea of having blood pressure measured in an office or hospital makes many patients sufficiently nervous to drive their blood pressures up higher than they would have been if taken by themselves at home. For this reason, as well as the vagaries in the equipment that is used, blood pressures frequently are taken more than once during a single office visit.

Translating Results of Medical Tests
into Diagnostic Decisions ....

■FROM PROBABILITIES TO DICHOTOMOUS ACTION

As has been shown in preceding sections of this chapter, sometimes a diagnosis is certain, as when direct evidence of a disease is observed, e.g., adenocarcinoma cells are visualized from a biopsy specimen of the colon. In other instances, a diagnosis is made using tests that yield only a probability that a disease is present in a particular patient. The usefulness of predictive values is that they assist in estimating the probability with which a disease is present or absent.

In order to decide to make a diagnosis, and to begin treatment, how large a probability (positive predictive value) is necessary? In order to decide that a patient is disease-free, and to withhold treatment, how large a probability (negative predictive value) is necessary?

There are no clear answers to these questions, no "cut-off" numbers that can be applied to all cases or all diseases. The reason for this is that different situations present different trade-offs, or different risk-benefit ratios. The predictive values for Lyme disease are not very high, largely because existing tests are not highly sensitive or specific. However, settling on a diagnosis of Lyme disease on the basis of a low positive predictive value would lead to a course of treatment with antibiotics which, at its worst, would be ineffective. In other words, there is relatively little in terms of health to be lost by treating a patient for Lyme disease. (On the other hand, failing to treat could permit the disease to progress to more debilitating and untreatable stages.)

Consider a dramatically different example: Several decades ago, a previously healthy clergyman began to show bizarre behavior, including disordered thinking and inability to function in his position. Psychiatric testing, sensitive for certain psychiatric disorders, diagnosed the patient as severely psychotic. His inability to function resulted in placement in a mental institution. Many years later, a physician examining the patient for general health recognized abnormal liver enzymes in the patient's blood work. The physician changed the diagnosis to a form of liver disease, ordering restriction of protein in the diet in lieu of psychotropic medications. Literally within days, the patient's behavior returned to normal. He was released from the mental institution without relapse, with a relatively simple regimen of controlled protein intake as his sole therapy. In this instance, hepatic encephalopathy was not considered in the differential diagnosis. The psychiatric tests that were performed were sensitive but not specific. Given a low specificity, the predictive value positive was also low—suggesting that a diagnosis of psychosis was being made with great uncertainty. The result of accepting a low predictive value to make a diagnosis resulted in the unnecessary "loss" of years of an individual's life.

Many examples could be provided to illustrate the difficulties involved in translating the results of medical tests and the probabilities of disease that can be calculated from test results, into "yes" (disease present) and "no" (disease absent) answers. Although there are no "rules-of-thumb" for what constitutes a "yes" versus a "no" answer to diagnostic questions, there are some considerations that can be helpful in using predictive values:

1. When a disease is potentially life threatening, and when timely treatment is of the essence in order to achieve a cure, relatively low probability of disease may be sufficient to initiate further action. For instance, a minority of the many women with abnormal mammograms who are sent for surgical biopsies actually have breast cancer. However, in those women with cancer, early detection and treatment can make the difference between complete cure and early mortality.

2. When a diagnostic test is itself risky, e.g., liver biopsy to confirm the diagnosis of hemochromatosis, and results of the test will have little or no impact on the treatment

of the disease, even a test with high predictive values might not be worth doing.

3. When a test is known to have high predictive values and is not terribly risky, but the disease in question is self-limiting or does not require treatment, it is reasonable to forego the discomfort, expense, and inconvenience of the test. For instance, young adult patients with complaints of common upper-respiratory symptoms during the winter (e.g., colds and flu), probably do not need arterial blood gases evaluated, unless symptoms of respiratory distress exacerbate, suggesting more serious pulmonary conditions.

In summary, higher positive or negative predictive values permit the physician to make a diagnosis of disease present or disease absent with greater certainty. Lower predictive values provide weaker evidence for presence or absence of disease. On the other hand, sometimes tests known to have low positive predictive values, such as mammograms, are used to initiate further action because missing a possible disease could have devastating results. These low predictive values can be due to low background prevalences. Conversely, sometimes tests known to have high predictive values, such as liver biopsy, are not used because the risks of the test outweigh the benefits to the patient in terms of medical treatment decisions.

To weigh complex risks and benefits involved in diagnostic testing, the technique of **decision analysis** can be extremely useful. Decision analysis is discussed in detail in Chapter 6 on Making Treatment Decisions and Prognostic Judgments, since it is most commonly used in treatment dilemmas.

■WHEN UNCERTAINTY REMAINS: NO HORSES OR ZEBRAS

In the health professions, there are a substantial number of times in which a diagnosis simply remains elusive and working diagnoses/hypotheses fail to result in a final diagnosis. This occurs rather frequently in an area of health care which might seem surprising to individuals who are not professionals in the particular field.

Two diseases that universally afflict humankind are dental caries (cavities) and periodontal (gum) disease. Included under this rubric are abscesses and infected pulps (necessitating root canals). The oral cavity is anatomically complex with a rich distribution of nerves, blood vessels, muscles, sinuses, teeth, and bone, all of which can be a source of mild to remarkably severe pain.

The differential diagnosis of oral pain can be straightforward or extremely elusive. Typically, a patient's chief complaint to a dentist will be a "toothache." During the dental history, the diagnostician will elicit descriptions of the type, duration, and patient's perception of location of the pain. Here, however, is a source of diagnostic difficulty.

Pain from the nerves located in the pulp chambers of teeth do not provide good information (sensory input to the patient) about the exact position of the tooth causing pain. In fact, the patient may not be able accurately to locate even the arch, maxillary, or mandibular, from which the pain emanates. This is because the pain signal from the tooth travels into the rich plexus of nerves of the face; and the pain may be perceived to be in a different, referred location in the mouth other than the site of the disease. Using X-ray films to detect endodontic problems is not always useful. Furthermore, not only can referred pain from impacted or abscessed teeth be present distant from the source of the pain, but also pain from other parts of the body can be perceived initially as dental pain. One of the first symptoms of a heart attack is sometimes pain in the lower jaw that feels very much like a toothache!

As in clinical medicine, dental tests of varying degrees of sensitivity, specificity, and predictive values exist to help arrive at a diagnosis and to remove the cause of the pain. However, when tests in medicine or dentistry fail to achieve a diagnosis, even by exclusion, empiric therapy may be the only solution. **Empiric therapy** is therapy given without strong evidence of disease, with the anticipation that if the diagnostic "hunch" is correct, the patient will respond favorably, thereby establishing that the hunch was the correct diagnosis (a somewhat backward way of reasoning compared with a typical differential!). Two possible forms of empiric therapy for toothache are extracting the suspicious tooth or opening it for treatment.

It is important to note that empiric therapy tends to be a poor vehicle for diagnosis, since any "resulting" improvements might be coincidental in the natural course of another disease (e.g., temporary cessation of cardiac-induced pain in unstable angina) or even a placebo effect of the intervention.

Summary

The ultimate endpoint sought by both patients and their physicians in the diagnostic process is an answer to the question of whether the patient has a particular disease. Between the question asked and the answer given lies a complex process that involves generating a working diagnosis based on the patient's symptoms and chief complaint, consideration of the patient's medical history, generating a differential diagnosis, testing the differential through the use of medical tests in addition to the medical history, and interpreting test results, which usually yield probabilities that a disease is present or absent. Medical tests used in the diagnostic process typically fall into two categories: Those used to rule in disease and those used to rule out disease. Concepts of sensitivity, specificity, and positive and negative predictive values comprise probabilities that assist the diagnostician to determine the likelihood that a patient has a disease or not. Based on complex information, and often without clear rules of thumb, the diagnostician attempts to arrive at a final diagnosis. When the typical process of making a diagnosis fails, a final alternative may be empiric therapy, that is, treating a possible disease with the expectation that favorable results will assist in establishing a correct diagnosis.

Suggested References ....

Ford, R.D. (Ed.). (1992). *Diagnostic tests handbook.* Springhouse, PA: Springhouse Publications. This handbook is a technical reference to nine different types of diagnostic testing. More than 450 diagnostic tests are covered, ranging from routine blood work to specialized cytologic tests and imaging techniques. For each test, the following information is provided: purpose, normal results, abnormal results, as well as relevant points about physiologic parameters and precautions for accuracy and safety.

Riegelman, R.K. (1991). *Minimizing medical mistakes: The art of medical decision making.* Boston: Little, Brown and Company. This book focuses primarily on making diagnostic decisions. It provides a particular approach to differential diagnosis that is easy to follow and accessible for both physicians and nonphysicians. It gives brief coverage to therapeutic decision-making (references for which are provided in the next chapter of this book).

Shtasel, P. (1991). *Medical tests and diagnostic procedures: A patient's guide to just what the doctor ordered.* New York: Harper Perennial. Sixteen areas of medical and surgical subspecialty are covered in this book, as well as five particular areas of imaging and laboratory tests: routine lab work, X-rays, nuclear studies, ultrasounds, and magnetic resonance imaging. The most common tests ordered in each of the 16 subspecialty areas covered in this book are described in lay terms. For each test a discomfort score and a hazard score are given. In addition, information about required hospital stays and pretest preparation is provided. While the discomfort and hazard scores are subjective and, having had some of the tests, one might quibble with the ratings, they are not terribly off course, and could probably be as useful to those ordering the tests as well as those undergoing them!

5

Chapter Five

Assessing the Health of Populations

Health is a state of complete physical, mental and social
well-being, not merely the absence of disease or infirmity.
World Health Organization

Introduction

In most of health care practice, the individual person is the patient who undergoes diagnostic testing and medical treatments.
When we consider health issues on a broader scale, the population rather than the individual is the "patient."

Obtaining accurate diagnostic information about a population
and "treating" a population fall under the responsibilities of public
health departments, which may serve the populations of cities,
states, countries, or even groups of countries. These departments
may range from local (e.g., municipal) health departments to
something as global as the World Health Organization.

For these organizations to function optimally, they must
have access to good information about the public health (and
illness) in their jurisdictions, as well as an understanding of how
best to use this information in developing public health policy.

Consequently, assessing the health of populations requires
a good understanding of some particular types of medical information.

■HEALTH, PUBLIC HEALTH, AND EPIDEMIOLOGY

The definition of health adopted by the World Health Organization (WHO) with which this chapter begins, presents a contemporary concept of health as not simply the absence of disease, but rather a more comprehensive state of overall well-being. Going even beyond that definition, the WHO recently has "experimented" with new ways of measuring quality of health care across countries, including in their measures the concepts of goodness and fairness of care (World Health Organization, 2000).

Historically, however, efforts to improve the health of groups of people, usually termed public health, has arisen from the need to control, treat, and eliminate disease. On the other hand, the wider view of health stated by WHO has lead public health research into areas not usually associated with disease. For example, rates of injury and death sustained in automobile accidents have been reduced by requiring the use of automobile seat belts.

In order to serve better the interests of public health, the field of epidemiology emerged. The most fundamental concerns of epidemiology have been the frequency of disease in humans, as well as its causes and geographical distributions.

Knowing the **burden of a disease** in a population, i.e., its frequency, provides indirect information about health by providing information about its opposite, illness. If it is possible to determine the causes of a particular disease, it may be possible to provide direction regarding treatment, or at least direction regarding the kinds of clinical research that might result in the discovery of effective treatments or cures. Tracking the geographical distribution of a disease can yield information about environmental and psychosocial risks, which may provide positive directions for eradication of disease. Tracking also alerts health departments to areas in need of assistance and provides individuals guidance about the relative safety, from a health perspective, of traveling to or living in particular locations.

In short, assessing the health of populations is an ongoing diagnostic process that assists in establishing the extent of certain diseases in given populations. However, rather than focus on the disease or well-being of one individual, this process is aimed at a meta-level view of the health of a village, community, country, or other subgroup of individuals. Social scientists, including medical anthropologists, continue to work with public health specialists and epidemiologists to arrive at strategies that will encompass a broader definition of health and the broader goal embraced by the WHO.

In spite of these intentions, during the last quarter of the twentieth century, the optimistic goal of enhancing health was somewhat eclipsed as world health was threatened by the emergence of such serious diseases as infection with human immunodeficiency virus (HIV) and Ebola Zaire, as well as upswings in both typical and multiple drug resistant strains of tuberculosis (TB and MDR-TB). In addition, breast cancer rates appear to be increasing among some populations of women; and many parts of the world are experiencing a decline in fertility rates, a phenomenon which is as yet poorly understood.

Assessing the health of populations continues to mandate attention to the frequency, causes, and geographical distributions of diseases, in order to provide direction to the clinicians, biochemists, and other scientists who are addressing emerging problems. In summary, assessing the health of populations continues to consist primarily of the tasks of diagnosing the pervasiveness and the seriousness of disease, and providing directions for implementing strategies that will enhance health and eradicate disease.

■COMMUNICABLE VERSUS NONCOMMUNICABLE DISEASES

Infectious disease epidemics and pandemics have occurred throughout human history. Progress in medical science has made us less vulnerable to their devastation now than at any point in the past. Nevertheless, the nation's current experience with human immunodeficiency virus (HIV) and ac-

quired immunodeficiency syndrome (AIDS) is a sobering re-
minder that serious microbial threats to health remain and
that we are not always well equipped to respond to them.

U. S. Institute of Medicine

The most devastating communicable disease outbreak recorded in human history was probably the outbreak of bubonic
plague that occurred during the Middle Ages. It has been estimated that within a time span of only 4 years, bubonic plague
resulted in the deaths of 25 million people in western Europe—
approximately one quarter of the population of the area at that
time.

Bubonic plague remains a highly fatal, infectious disease
that still occurs in several areas of the world, including (but only
rarely) western areas of the United States. Study of plague transmission revealed that the primary disease reservoir is an infected
wild rodent, and transmission to humans is through the bite of infected fleas, which are the primary disease vector. Pneumonic
plague may occur as a result of contact, direct or droplet, with another person with bubonic plague or as primary pneumonic
plague, both of which are air-borne and highly transmissible from
person to person, i.e., communicable.

More recent examples of infectious (communicable) diseases include Ebola Zaire and hantaviruses. In 1976, an outbreak of a hemorrhagic fever later named Ebola Zaire decimated
some villages in Zaire and the Sudan. While the outbreaks occurred in relatively isolated sites, and transmission beyond the
villages was minimal, the mortality rate was an astounding 75%
in those who were infected. In 1993, 16 individuals living on or
near a Navaho reservation in the southeastern United States developed and died from a flu-like illness, which was tentatively
attributed to some form of hantavirus, which is known to cause
lethal fevers in parts of Asia.

In the United States, there are diseases that are considered
to be "reportable" meaning that they must be reported to the
Centers for Disease Control and Prevention (CDC) by physicians, hospitals, and state health agencies. These are all infec-

tious diseases that require quarantine in order to halt the spread of disease and include: cholera, diphtheria, plague, smallpox, most forms of tuberculosis, viral hemorrhagic fevers, and yellow fever. In the United States, chronic, noncommunicable diseases are not "reportable" so it is more difficult to obtain information about their pervasiveness in the population.

Reporting instances of disease typically is termed **surveillance** or, more rarely, medical intelligence. The purpose of gathering public health information of this kind is to identify where and when outbreaks of diseases are occurring and to mobilize public health resources and medical facilities to cope with the outbreaks. Surveillance can be divided into active and passive forms. Active surveillance occurs when health care professionals such as epidemiologists and infection control specialists take an active role in data gathering, as in tracking down contacts of infectious cases. Active surveillance often requires going into the community in which the index case has lived or worked. (An index case is a primary case of an infectious disease from which links to other cases may be traced.) Passive surveillance is the form of information gathering that occurs through reportable diseases, i.e., when required data are submitted to a central location by the sites covered by the surveillance program. In the State of Connecticut, all tumors found by health care professionals across all health care sites are reportable to the Tumor Registry, which is a state-run, passive surveillance project.

While the CDC has placed a heavy emphasis on tracking communicable diseases (such as HIV and TB), full pictures of public health also must include diseases that are not believed to be infectious, including heart disease and cancer.

Tracking noncommunicable diseases serves some important functions. Consider, for example, the finding that more cases of breast cancer are being identified in some areas of the United States than in others and among some ethnic groups more than others. This tracking enables scientists not only to generate meta-level views of the breast health of women living in the United States, but also to investigate possible causes for higher rates of breast cancer in particular geographical areas or among particular ethnic groups. Finding at-risk subgroups of the population can lead to enhanced efforts at early ident-ification of disease and better outcomes from available treatments.

Some medical concerns, such as decreased fertility rates in many countries, may have complex explanations including en-vironmental factors, age at first attempted pregnancy, history of diseases related to infertility, etc. While causes are not suffi-ciently clear, the availability of fertility data permits researchers to derive comparisons of fertility rates over different points in time and across different countries, in order to arrive at the con-clusion that decreased fertility is an issue of concern among many contemporary populations.

Obtaining Data About the Health of Populations

If we believe that vaccination protects against the develop-ment of smallpox it is not because there has been a direct experimental demonstration but rather (a) there is a good deal of evidence that is consistent with this hypothesis, and (b) over the course of many years no evidence has been produced to support any alternative hypothesis. The truth of the matter appears to be that medical knowledge (and one suspects, many other kinds as well) has always advanced by a combination of many different kinds of observation, some controlled and some uncontrolled, some directly and some only tangentially relevant to the problems at hand . . .

Cornfield

■THE TERMS AND TOOLS OF EPIDEMIOLOGY

The field most closely associated with gathering information about the health of populations is epidemiology. The derivation of the word is "epi" meaning upon and "demic" from "demos" meaning the people, collectively. Thus, **epidemiology** focuses on those events (i.e., diseases) which have been visited upon the people.

Epidemiology borrows and adapts tools and methods from many sources including biology, clinical medicine, laboratory medicine, statistics and mathematical modeling, social science, and engineering. These tools and methods, combined with curiosity, persistence, keen observation of human behavior, copious notes, and the use of what is termed "shoe leather" to track down and document events, have produced impressive results in the prevention and control of disease. Public health information is thought of as surveillance data, and the epidemiologist often plays a kind of detective's role in obtaining it.

The role of the epidemiologist typically is to develop a factually and temporally precise statement of the occurrence of an event, which may be an infectious process or a physiologic abnormality in the population. While epidemiology has developed largely from attempts to understand and control infectious processes, it is not limited to this focus.

Occurrences of disease are classified as being sporadic, endemic, epidemic, pandemic, or not of infectious origin. **Sporadic** events usually are point-source outbreaks that occur from time to time. An outbreak of multiple drug resistant TB in an isolated Inuit village is sporadic. **Endemic** means that a particular disease is pervasive, usually referring to a part of the world in which large segments of the population have the disease. For example, infection with tuberculosis is endemic in many if not most developing countries. **Epidemic** and **pandemic** refer to mass contagions in which numbers of cases continue to increase until effective treatment for the disease is discovered or all susceptible individuals have become infected. Epidemics refer to large geographical areas; pandemics refer to the world. HIV infection was first thought to be epidemic in the United States. Recent trends show that HIV has appeared across many countries and continents and, as a global threat, is now pandemic. The last pandemic was the influenza outbreak of 1918, which resulted in astounding mortality rates on multiple continents.

The terms introduced above all refer to infectious (communicable) diseases and the result of a parasite gaining entry into a host. Diseases that are not infectious but may be of concern to epidemiologists can result from such varied causes as environmental contamination, radiation, addiction, accident, and trauma.

The impact of diseases on the population are reported by epidemiologists in several ways:

- A **rate** is a measure of occurrence over time. **Mortality rate** is a measure of the number of deaths that have occurred over time and are attributed to particular causes. For example, mortality rates are reported for HIV disease and for TB. **Morbidity rate** is a measure of incapacitation over time. Morbidity rates associated with lower back injuries are reported for use by insurance companies and workmen's compensation boards. **Prevalence rate** is the proportion of people who have a disease at a given point in time, taking into account everyone who is living who has been diagnosed with the disease. An estimate of prevalence rate for breast cancer among U.S. women as of 2001 is 1 in 8. **Incidence rate** is a measure of numbers of new cases occurring, usually on a yearly basis. New, or incident, cases of breast cancer are tallied each year in attempts to find out whether this disease is increasing, decreasing, or remaining stable among U.S. women. (See Chapter 4 on Generating Diagnoses for more information about how to calculate incidence and prevalence rates.)
- **Risk** is the probability that a disease will occur within a specific time period. The risk of developing active TB after becoming infected with the bacillus has been estimated to range from 2 to 10% in persons who are not immune-compromised. **Risk factors** refer to conditions or states present in a population that are believed to be related to the occurrence of the disease. For example,

individuals infected with HIV are at greater risk for developing active TB than individuals who are HIV-seronegative. Women with strong family histories of breast cancer, such as breast cancer in first-degree relatives, are at higher risk for developing breast cancer than the general population.

- **Surveillance** is the ongoing active and passive observation and reporting, often mandatory, of the status of diseases within a population. In the United States, sexually transmitted diseases such as syphilis must be reported by the treating physician to the appropriate public health authority.
- **Screening** refers to the use of diagnostic tests on a broad scale to determine the presence of a condition in a population who are asymptomatic or have not been diagnosed at that time. In the United States, mass screenings for hypertension are often conducted in public sites such as shopping malls. In Canada, anonymous screening sites for HIV disease have been set up in many major cities.
- **Vital statistics** are comprised of information collected about major life events, such as date of birth, ethnicity, parents, marriage, divorce, death, and cause of death. These statistics can provide important background information on a population that is being studied.

■GOALS OF EPIDEMIOLOGICAL RESEARCH

There are four general goals or phases of epidemiological research and three general questions that usually frame the research. These are listed below, with reminders that the population rather than the individual is the unit of study.

Epidemiology targets three major questions:

1. Which kind of disease or diseases does the patient [population] have?

2. Which kind of patient [population] does the disease have, i.e., which characteristics of the population, such as risk factors, might be important to know?
3. What is the cultural perspective of the disease, i.e., how is it understood and thought about in relevant populations?

The four phases of epidemiological research are descriptive, constructive, experimental, and evaluative (relating to implementation of public health programs).

Descriptive epidemiology asks:

1. What is the nature of the event, i.e., what specifically has happened?
2. Which groups in the population were affected?
3. When and over what period of time did the effect occur?
4. Where and over what spatial area did the effect occur?
5. Under what set of circumstances did the effect occur?

Constructive epidemiology begins the process of attempting to construct meaning from descriptive information. Constructive epidemiology asks:

1. Why did the event occur?
2. How can such events be prevented?

Experimental epidemiology attempts to find out whether our understanding of what has occurred is correct. To accomplish this task, experimental investigations are necessary. Experimental epidemiology is characterized by the questions:

1. Which hypotheses can and should be tested?
2. Which preventive measures can be used effectively to prevent the disease?

Implementation is the final phase, in which programs that have been developed from a research base are put into practice for the prevention and control of disease. **Evaluation research** is conducted to determine:

1. Is implementation of the intervention feasible as planned?
2. To what extent has the intervention program accomplished its goals?

The ultimate objective of epidemiological studies is to develop rational and practical plans for the prevention and control of the event. Complete elimination of disease is desirable but not usually possible or feasible. Smallpox appears to be the only infectious disease that has been eliminated as a result of a concerted effort worldwide to vaccinate all susceptible populations. While once endemic in many areas, the last case of smallpox was reported in 1973. The last remaining smallpox virus is stored in freezers in research laboratories. A plan to eliminate tuberculosis in the United States by 2000 did not progress on schedule. Instead, increasing rates of HIV infection during the last decades of the twentieth century along with the emergence of multiple drug resistant strains of tuberculosis, contributed to an increase in TB in many areas. The Centers for Disease Control and Prevention (CDC) continues to work out recommendations for the prevention of HIV and TB (American Thoracic Society/Centers for Disease Control Statement Committee on Latent Tuberculosis Infection, 2000).

Epidemiologists view disease from both biological and social perspectives during their investigations. Snow (1855), in his investigation of the cholera epidemic in 1850s London, mapped deaths from cholera, delivery of water by water company, and source of water by well pump. Based on these observations, he was able to identify a water source that was associated with high death rates and took action to have the well closed. In another instance, epidemiologists, called in to investigate a number of deaths in a small village, were given the explanation that the deaths were a result of poor sanitation. However, one epidemiologist observed that bags of seed grain stored in a shed had been opened. That grain had been given to the village to help them replant and recover from a period of poor crops. The seed grain had been treated with an antifungal agent to permit it to be stored until time to replant. The antifungal agent contained a mercury compound that was toxic if ingested. As a result of famine in the village, some of this grain intended only for planting had been stolen and eaten, resulting in mercury poisoning and deaths. Consequently, the reported mortalities resulted not from poor sanitation but rather from famine-related ingestion of a toxic substance.

Counting and observing remain basic epidemiological tools. Even in this age of information in cyberspace, good epidemiological studies do not necessarily require high-tech microcomputers and sophisticated statistical techniques to produce results.

■FLUORIDATION: AN EXAMPLE OF A CLASSIC EPIDEMIOLOGICAL INVESTIGATION

What follows is a detailed account of a well-known epidemiological investigation that resulted in a somewhat controversial recommendation to fluoridate public water supplies. The investigation is divided into stages corresponding to those discussed above.

The Descriptive Phase

In 1902, Dr. Fred McKay, a dentist, moved from the northeastern United States to Colorado where he established a dental practice. Dr. McKay observed that many of his new patients in Colorado had a permanent discoloration of the enamel of their teeth, which he named "Colorado brown stain." He had not noticed this type of intrinsic stain of enamel in his patients in the northeast and began a lifetime effort to determine the nature of the stain. The stain caused no discomfort, apparently was not contagious, and was not a result of dental caries (tooth decay), or any other known disease of the teeth.

McKay perceived the stain to be solely a cosmetic problem that could become sufficiently severe to result in mottling and pitting of the enamel. At the time, his patients did not seem to perceive the stain as a cosmetic problem, probably because so many in their community had teeth with the same stain. McKay spent his free time and his own money investigating the stain, traveling locally, statewide, and ultimately worldwide to investigate reports of similar conditions. He determined that 87% of the children native to his region of Colorado developed the stain to some degree, but that people who moved to the area after childhood did not develop the condition. He discovered also that this condition existed in other parts of the United States and in other parts of the world.

For 22 years he worked alone in his spare time documenting and charting the occurrence of the condition. He contacted respected experts in dentistry and in the development of enamel who expressed little interest in his efforts except to remark that is was strange that a dental lesion endemic to many regions and affecting so many people would be unreported in the dental literature. Many changes were occurring in the United States at this time. People began to leave their home towns to go to school, and many began to travel more widely. At the same time, smiles became a mark of success and attractiveness in advertisements and movies. These social changes suggested that the Colorado brown stain would soon become a source of concern.

The Constructive Phase

McKay sought to understand this condition in order to control or eliminate the defect. His primary question was whether "something in the local water caused the condition." He also observed paradoxically that "the most poorly calcified enamel was the least susceptible to dental caries."

He had hundreds of water samples tested chemically to determine if there were any differences between the water supplies in the endemic areas versus stain-free areas. No chemical test of that time (1902–1928) detected any consistent difference in the water samples that would explain the presence of the stain. His observation concerning the resistance of the stained enamel to dental caries met with strong criticism from leaders in the health professions of the time. Authorities in the field believed that well-mineralized, "white" teeth were strong and desirable. Large sums of advertising money were spent advising people to "drink milk to build strong bones and teeth."

However, one community, Oakley, Idaho, listened to McKay. Every child who was born and grew up in Oakley drinking the city well water had severely mottled enamel. In 1925, after consulting with McKay, the parents in Oakley agreed to dig another well in a different area in the hope that changing the water source would prevent mottling of the enamel. Seven years later, when the permanent teeth erupted in the children who drank the changed water supply, there were no stains. (Of course, this new site for the water source was a lucky choice, since McKay could not have made tests to determine whether the water at the new site was in fact different from the original water supply.)

At approximately the same time, the Aluminum Company of America (ALCOA) built a company town in Bauxite, Arkansas. They made, among other products, a new type of aluminum cooking utensils which they had begun marketing. There was resistance to these utensils because it was claimed that they could poison you if you used them to cook. At the same time, it was discovered that the children in Bauxite had stained and mottled teeth which alarmed ALCOA because it might give credence to the claim that there was harm in using aluminum cooking utensils. Consequently, in 1930 an ALCOA chemist analyzed the water from Bauxite. Using the technique of spectrography, a high and unexpected amount of the element fluorine (13.7 parts per million) was identified. McKay sent water to be tested from endemic areas, all of which showed high concentrations of fluorine, from 2 to 13 (parts per million). Concurrently, another research team, unaware of the work at ALCOA, had shown that rats fed diets high in fluoride developed mottled enamel. Thus, an animal model and a human model appeared at the same time. The fluoride-water connection to stain and mottling was demonstrated, thereby validating McKays' 30 years of work.

The observation that tooth enamel formed in areas where the water supply was high in fluoride might also be resistant to dental caries became the focus of detailed investigation that continues today. Interest in dental health, and the scientific approach to the study of dental disease, progressed in parallel to growth in general medical science during the twentieth century. Dental caries (decay) and periodontal problems (gum disease), were the most widespread of all diseases. The pain and infection associated with abscessed teeth and infected gums, while not often fatal, resulted in high morbidity (loss of work, poor general health) in the society of the 1930s prior to the advent of antibiotics to treat oral infections and when most of the techniques for local anesthesia and diagnostic radiology were still being developed.

During World War I, the morbidity for a severe oral infection called "trench mouth" resulted in more soldiers being hospitalized than did battlefield wounds. Tooth loss from decay and gum disease kept many individuals out of the armed forces altogether, since there was a requirement that recruits needed sufficient teeth to "masticate the basic army ration." At that time, a significant number of young men had fewer than seven natural teeth in their mouths that could be used to masticate. In 1931 a request was made to the Public Health Service (PHS) that a dental surgeon be assigned to follow up the role of fluoride in dental health. The PHS assigned H. Trendly Dean to the investigation.

Dean began a systematic investigation of the brown stain phenomenon, much of which was conducted by going from door to door asking questions (a "shoe leather" survey.) Another extensive survey using questionnaires was conducted targeting every dental society in the United States. By 1936, Dean had documented that at 1 ppm of fluoride in the water, less than 10% of the population had mottling in even its mildest form. His next step was an investigation of the relation between mottling, fluoride, and decay. Using data he collected on decayed teeth in areas with and without mottling, he was able to document that mottled teeth were decay resistant.

The Experimental Phase

Dean and his colleague, F. A. Arnold, began a large-scale controlled study involving 21 cities with varying amounts of fluoride in the water, but similar in terms of racial and ethnic composition, amounts of sunlight, and the same mineral composition of the water. The cities varied in population size and in geographic location. Over a 2-year period, the researchers conducted dental examinations of over 7000 school children between the ages of 12 and 14. At the conclusion of the study, in 1943, they reported that the cities with the lowest fluoride content in the water had the highest rate of decay, and that the city with the highest concentration of fluoride had the lowest rate of decay. Also, at 1 ppm of fluoride there was strikingly little decay and only sporadic incidences of the mildest form of mottling (now called fluorosis).

Investigations into the physiological effects of fluoride in humans began at about the same time as the work of Dean and Arnold. The concern that fluoride was known to be toxic at higher concentrations could not be dismissed without study. After hundreds of studies there was no evidence for deleterious effects of low levels of fluoride on any other aspect of health. In fact, it appeared that fluoride was associated with fewer fractures in older women, which indicated that fluoride might reduce osteoporosis.

Finally, the fluoride-decay hypothesis was subjected to a rigorous experimental test. The hypothesis was that raising the concentration of fluoride in water to 1 ppm should result in a reduction in dental caries and not result in fluorosis, nor in any other reduction in the general health of the population. In 1945, several pairs of cities were selected to participate in the experimental study. Using the same methods developed in the study of 21 cities, baseline data were collected including dental and health records. Data collection continued for the next 15 years. Results showed that all the control cities had higher rates of tooth decay than did the cities with fluoride in the water supplies. After the initial results were made public, most of the control cities elected to add fluoride to their water supply before the end of the 15 years. Similar studies were conducted worldwide with similar results. Data now exist that document 50+ years of success for fluoridation of public water supplies.

The Implementation Phase

There continues to be controversy concerning the fluoridation of public water supplies. These controversies focus on the following issues and opinions:

1. No reasonable relationship exists between fluoridation and the maintenance of public health.
2. The prevention of dental decay is not a proper objective of joint community effort.
3. Fluoridation cannot be legally authorized by a community.
4. Fluoridation violates constitutional rights (such as religious freedom to reject medical interventions).
5. Fluoridation represents the unlicensed practice of medicine, dentistry, and pharmacy.
6. There are many health risks associated with the "mass medication" of public water supplies.

The legal questions relating to these controversies and the "police power" of public health officials in society have been resolved regarding fluoridation in the courts: Fluoridation of community water supplies that have been judged to be deficient in fluoride can legally be supplemented to eliminate this deficiency. The health risk questions have been investigated in detail, and no association with health risk and water fluoridation at the recommended level have been found. Major health agencies and professional health associations worldwide endorse fluoridation and state that the opponents of fluoridation have been discredited.

Nevertheless, a history of resistance to fluoridation persists. "A dentist representing the American Dental Association noted in the House subcommittee hearing . . . (that) 'Fluoridation may well be the most thoroughly studied community health measure of recent history.'" Fluoridation of community water supplies is one of the few public health measures that is voted upon in public elections. It is the overwhelming opinion of the scientific community, according to a World Health Organization report issued in 1970, that "the only sign of physiological or pathological change in life-long users of optimally fluoridated water supplies . . . is that they suffer less from tooth decay." Informed scientific opinion notwithstanding, hundreds of communities have voted down water fluoridation, or, in some cases, voted to stop fluoridation that had been implemented at an earlier time. At present, somewhat more than 50% of the population of the United States drink fluoridated water. "About 100 million Americans do not, largely because of the fears raised by opponents of fluoridation. The simple truth is that there is no 'scientific controversy' over the safety of fluoridation. The practice is safe, economical, and beneficial. The survival of this fake controversy represents . . . one of the major triumphs of quackery over science in our generation" (Consumers Reports, 1978a, 1978b).

Good data and good recommendations do not automatically result in the implementation of informed public policy. Political reality, social, legal, and ethical issues must always be addressed when decisions impacting on the health and welfare of the public are concerned. Data are only a part of the process leading to implementation of public policy decisions.

■SURVEY RESEARCH: THE PRIMARY INVESTIGATIVE METHOD OF EPIDEMIOLOGY

Field Surveys Used to Generate an Index

Surveys of large populations may be undertaken to establish an index of health or disease. An **index** is a ratio of the number of individuals who have a given disease or condition to the total number of individuals in the target population. The index is used to describe mathematically the health status of a population.

An index typically is obtained from **field research** in which investigators make observations of large samples of people, often under difficult conditions. To be useful, an index must be:

- *Quantitative.* Expressed in meaningful numerical terms, it must be amenable to test by professional and statistical logic. An index is a numerical value describing the relative status of a population on a graduated scale with definite upper and lower limits designed to permit and facilitate comparison with other populations classified by the same criteria and methods.
- *Simple, usable, and inexpensive.* An index should be simple so that it can be used quickly in large population groups. It should be inexpensive, efficient, require little or no equipment, and be inoffensive and acceptable to the individual patient and to the target group's social and cultural values.
- *Reproducible.* Reproduciblity or reliability permits similar results to be obtained by different examiners. If an index is reproducible, results from one study can be compared with results from other studies.
- *Valid.* The index must measure the condition it purports to measure, and measure it across population and environmental differences.
- *Criterion-based.* Criteria for identifying or diagnosing a disease or condition must be carefully and unambiguously stated. The criteria must be adhered to carefully to assure reproducibility and validity. Examiners who use the index should require little training to obtain the information necessary for the index.

Dean and Arnold used several indexes in their fluoridation study. They developed an index of the degree of fluorosis of teeth and an index for dental caries. The dental caries index is widely used and can serve as an example: **DMF index**—The letters D, M, and F refer to a cumulative lifetime experience of the number of "decayed," "missing," and "filled," permanent teeth. The unit of measurement can be teeth or individual surfaces of each tooth; in the latter case the index is reported as a DMFS. A population is examined, and the total number of DMF teeth is obtained for each age group. This total is divided by the number of individuals in the group to obtain the DMF teeth per person at that age.

Questionnaire-Based Surveys

Questionnaires often are used to obtain public health data and frequently serve as part of a larger project that also requires collection of clinical data. Usually questionnaires are constructed to collect demographic information, attitudes and opinions, or facts related to delivery of health services.

The primary methodological issues in survey research are as follows:

- *From whom should data be collected?* In other words, the target population must be defined carefully. Since it is unlikely that all members of even a small population will be approached for study, defining the target group involves complex problems of sampling.
- *Which is the optimal method to use to collect the information?* Surveys may be mailed or done by telephone or door-to-door. (Additionally, surveys can be conducted via computer when sufficient numbers of target participants are available online.) Each method has its particular drawbacks. For example, if a telephone survey is done, individuals who do not have telephones in their homes will be excluded from the survey, creating a systematic bias in the data.
- *How should the data be analyzed and interpreted?* Survey research using questionnaires typically does not lend itself to inferential statistics. The analytic methods of choice are typically descriptive statistics, such as frequencies and percentages, with careful attention paid to such potential sources of bias as missing data occurring systematically on a particular question.

Using Data About Public Health ....

■GOVERNANCE, PUBLIC HEALTH, AND SAFETY

Public health officials, offices, and services are found in all levels of government: federal, state, county, and city. Physicians, nurses, dentists, health inspectors, veterinarians, and sanitation engineers, among others, are charged with overseeing the many aspects of our day-to-day life that impact on health and public safety. Everything from routine treatment of drinking water to field investigations of suspected outbreaks of an infectious disease come under the responsibilities of health agencies and departments. Public health laws give health officers broad powers to protect the health of the public. Quarantine and closure of unsanitary food preparation sites are within the police power of health officials. Justice Harlan, in an opinion on the validity of a statute on vaccination, stated that "according to settled principles, the police power of a State must be held to embrace, at least, such reasonable regulations established directly by legislative enactment as will protect the public health and public safety" (Maier, 1963, p. 33). Many public health measures are part of law. Vaccinations before attending school and medical examination before employment as food handler are two examples.

Data are used to guide public health measures in two important instances:

- Making decisions on public policy and law
- Guiding individuals in seeking or using health services or measures

It is the responsibility of public health services to interpret relevant data, educate the public, and support policymakers in the implementation of effective public heath measures, as well as to monitor and revise these measures for the public good.

■BREAST CANCER: AN EXAMPLE OF THE USE OF PUBLIC HEALTH INFORMATION BY THE LAY PUBLIC

Nearly unlimited access to health information on the Internet has empowered the layperson to collect, question, and interpret public health data. (For extensive discussion of use of Internet information, see Chapter 7, Medical Information in Cyberspace.) While consumers who are not health professionals have access to these data, they may not be well prepared to understand the sophisticated ways in which public health data are framed and reported. An excellent example of the ways in which good public health data can be understood or misunderstood is contained in *The New England Journal of Medicine,* Putting the Risk of Breast Cancer in Perspective, January 14, 1999, Volume 340, Number 2, which explores the misconceptions about the relative risks of breast cancer. This section will use this report to illustrate the nature of public health information available regarding breast cancer and to highlight the areas in which medical information on breast cancer has been misunderstood. The quoted sections in the following discussion are from Phillips et al., 1999 (pp.1839–1840).

Breast cancer is not, by law, a reportable infectious disease, which means that no central agency collects nationwide data on breast cancer. Individual states or consortiums may have well-maintained tumor registries that may have collected masses of data on breast disease. These data sources typically are available for scientific research and may be accessible online to an interested layperson. There are also many agencies that publish information about the impact of breast cancer, its risk, early detection, and treatment, with an implied promise that lives will be saved if prompt and proper diagnosis and treatment are obtained. Breast cancer is a health problem that is constantly in the media, bringing its nature and consequences continually to the attention of the public. "However, for this information to be interpretable, it should be presented in a form that enables the risk to be understood in context. This is rarely the case, because of the difficulties involved in conveying

such inherently complex information to a population and to individual women.

Statistics from studies are quoted often to emphasize the
magnitude of the risk. "Several studies have shown that women
tend to overestimate their risk of breast cancer and that many
fail to understand the importance of age as a risk factor. The familiar "one in nine" statistic, much quoted in both the medical
literature and the media, refers to the cumulative lifetime risk of
breast cancer for a woman who lives past the age of 85." The 1
in 9 statistic has not, in fact, been constant. (Now, as of 2001,
the risk typically is reported as 1 in 8.) It had been reported as
1 in 11 for many years and then reported as 1 in 9 when the
age base of the population was adjusted from ending at age 70
to ending at age 85, effectively including more higher risk patients but representing no real increase in risk to any individual
patient. This change in risk, as it was reported in the popular
press, may have led some women to believe that a drastic increase in their personal risk of breast cancer had occurred for
some "unexplained" reason. This belief may be supported because "there is a common misconception that the yearly risk of
breast cancer remains relatively constant with age, leading
many younger women to view this statistic as a short-term
probability and grossly overestimate their risk of breast cancer
in a 10-year period."

The report continues with clear presentation of the difficulties faced by the layperson in obtaining a perspective on the
true risk of breast cancer in their life.

It is usually difficult to place risk estimates into a meaningful context. "A useful starting point for a discussion of the
risk of breast cancer is the 1-in-9 statistic. Although seemingly
easy to comprehend, this figure warrants closer scrutiny. Put in
context, it means that on average, for any group of 9 women,
breast cancer will develop in one of them at some time in her
life, but not in the remaining 8. The 1 woman in whom breast
cancer does develop has a 50% chance of receiving the diagnosis after the age of 65 and a 60% chance of surviving that
cancer and of dying from another cause. Because it is a cu-

mulative risk estimate, the 1-in-9 statistic, although accurate, is the most dramatic way of describing the risk. It was used by the American Cancer Society in campaigns in the early 1990s to improve compliance with mammographic screening programs. In fact, the risk of breast cancer for a woman in any given decade of her life never approaches 1 in 9. Breast cancer is uncommon at younger ages, so the risk in earlier decades is low . . . a woman entering her 30s has a 1 in 250 chance of breast cancer in the next 10 years. The risk of breast cancer increases with age, so that a woman entering her 40s has a 1 in 77 chance of the disease in the following decade. Breast cancer is much more common at older ages, but the risk of breast cancer in any given decade of life never exceeds 1 in 34. Included in the population on which these data are based, however, are subgroups of women who are at significantly higher risk for breast cancer, such as those with a strong family history of the disease."

The concept of mortality rate can be especially difficult to place into perspective when just one of a number of possible risks is discussed. "We are all exposed to multiple risks for various adverse events every day, although we are largely unaware of them. To gain perspective, we should consider the risk of death from breast cancer in the context of the competing risks of death from other diseases. The cause of death among women at any age is always more likely to be something other than breast cancer."

Misunderstanding the data regarding breast cancer risks can contribute to misinformed health choices on the part of consumers. Focus on breast cancer risks in the absence of a perspective on other types of risks can eclipse the importance of health behaviors that are associated with prevention of deaths from other causes. For example, a woman at low risk for breast cancer might elect to forego hormone replacement therapy (HRT) after menopause because she fears the possible increased risk of breast cancer that might be associated with HRT. In her concerns regarding breast cancer, she might ignore her risk for heart disease, and might not realize the possible cardiac benefits conferred by HRT. She might not ever understand that heart disease is the leading cause of death among women in the United States. Furthermore, she might not understand that among cancers, lung cancer rather than breast cancer is the leading cause of cancer deaths among women. Consequently, she might ignore the opportunity to quit smoking.

In addition, misconception of the risks of breast cancer—and, in particular, thinking the risks are much higher than they appear actually to be—can backfire in the campaigns for mass screenings. When individuals believe that a disease is extremely likely to occur, that it is all but a foregone conclusion, they might feel helpless and fearful. Such responses can act strongly as barriers rather than facilitators to adherence with a screening regimen.

In addition to the misinterpretations discussed above, other problems can emerge when using population data to predict individual risk (or benefit). A phenomenon called the **ecological fallacy** can occur when conclusions from large data sets are used to make estimates of an individual's personal risk. This means that data which represent "the greatest good for greatest numbers" might not provide the appropriate direction for the individual. The ecological fallacy can become especially problematic when the unit of analysis in the study is something other than the single case, as when cities or health care sites rather than individual patients are sampled and data are presented by city or site. In Chapter 3, Table 3c was presented illustrating the numbers of cases of HIV and AIDS by state. The number of cases in New York was much higher than the number for many other states. These numbers reflect the state as the unit of analysis; the findings do not mean that an individual in New York is at higher risk for HIV disease than an individual in Arkansas, for example. The numbers do mean that the burden of HIV disease is greater in New York than in many other states. Returning to the breast cancer issue, rates of breast cancer for women living on Long Island, NY, have been calculated as higher than those for women in other regions. Avoiding the ecological fallacy, this does not necessarily mean that a particular woman has a high risk for breast cancer and should, for example, avoid hormone replacement therapy simply because she resides on Long Island.

Summary

The field of public health focuses on the health of populations rather than the clinical care of individual patients. The population targeted by public health can be a village, community, state, country, or other geographic unit, including the world. The World Health Organization has been attempting to define health in larger terms than only the absence of disease.

Epidemiology is the study of disease in populations. The phases of epidemiological research are descriptive, constructive, experimental, and evaluative. The history of water fluoridation provides a good and complete example of the four phases of epidemiological research. Calculating morbidity, mortality, and risk rates also are tasks that fall within the domain of epidemiology. Data for these calculations often are obtained from survey research designed to develop indexes of disease in a population.

Infectious diseases are categorized as sporadic, endemic, epidemic, and pandemic. Information about infectious diseases may be obtained by health departments through the use of both active and passive surveillance. Public health also encompasses diseases that are not infectious, such as heart disease and cancer.

Since public health data typically are intended for use by policymakers at the level of the city, state, or some other geographic unit, the units of analysis may be inappropriate for making decisions about individual patients. Misunderstandings about the ways in which public health data should be used can result in inappropriate decisions for individuals. The example of breast cancer risks, with the slogan "1 in 9" is an instance in which the risk of this disease obtained from large samples over the course of lifetimes can be misinterpreted as the risk an individual woman who has not had breast cancer faces at any given moment in time. Misunderstandings of public health data can result in negative ramifications for both individual and public health, as when fear of extremely high likelihood of breast cancer creates fear and discourages women from adherence with screening recommendations.

Suggested References

Alreck, P.L., & Settle, R.B. (1995). *The survey research handbook.* New York, McGraw-Hill. A practical guide to survey research methods and applications. Comprehensive in scope without emphasis on statistics. The principles of planning and implementing a survey are presented in step-by-step detail.

Greenberg, R. S. (1993). *Medical epidemiology.* Norwalk, CT, Appleton & Lange. An introduction to epidemiology for medical, nursing, dental, pharmacy, and veterinary students. The text presents an overview of the role of epidemiology in medicine. It is not intended to be comprehensive. However, a survey of the basic methods used in epidemiological studies is presented with clear examples and study questions.

Citations in Text

American Thoracic Society/Centers for Disease Control and Prevention Statement Committee on Latent Tuberculosis Infection. (2000). Targeted tuberculin testing and treatment of latent tuberculosis infection. *Am. J. Respir. Crit. Care. Med., 161:4* (part 2).

Consumer Reports. (1978a) Fluoridation—The cancer scare—Part 1. *Consumer Reports,* July, 392–396.

Consumer Reports. (1978b) Six ways to mislead the public—The attack on fluoridation—Part 2. *Consumer Reports,* August, 480–482.

Maier, F.J. (1963). *Manual of water fluoridation practice.* New York, McGraw-Hill.

Phillips, K.A., Glendon, G. & Knight, J.A. (1999). Putting the risk of breast cancer in perspective. *N Eng J Med, 340 (2),* 1839–1840.

Snow, J. (1855). On the mode of communications of cholera (2nd. Ed.). London: Churchill.

World Health Organization. (2000). The World Health Report 2000—health systems: Improving performance. Geneva, Switzerland. World Health Organization Publications.

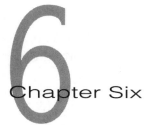

Chapter Six

Making Treatment Decisions and Prognostic Judgments

Above all, do no harm.

Hippocratic Oath

The value of life lies not in the length of days but in the use you make of them.

Michel Eyquem de Montaigne

Introduction

■ THE STARTING POINT: A CORRECT DIAGNOSIS

Deciding which medical therapy to use can involve many factors, the first of which is a correct diagnosis. This point may seem absurdly obvious. However, recall that medical reasoning can involve a significant amount of uncertainty, and that diagnostic conclusions often are no more than the best estimates physicians can make from probabilistic data.

Consider the example used previously in this text of the patient hospitalized with a diagnosis of psychosis and treated with psychotropic medications appropriate to this diagnosis. The patient's medical therapy may have been "optimal" given the choices of psychotropic drugs available at the time. However, the patient's condition was misdiagnosed: He suffered not from a primary psychiatric condition, but rather from a type of liver disease that interfered with the metabolism of protein, ultimately causing hepatic encephalopathy. With a correct diagnosis, the patient would have been treated best by a protein-restricted diet and no psychotropic medications.

It is difficult if not impossible to know how often medical therapies are thought to be at fault (ineffective) when, in fact, the problem is an incorrect diagnosis. Some disease entities are more likely than others to reveal their true nature over time. For example, if a case of systemic lupus erythematosis is misdiagnosed as chronic fatigue syndrome, at some point the characteristic lupus "butterfly" rash may appear, thus clinching a correction. Other diseases may never show clear signs of what they are, and even may be "masked" by inappropriate therapies. For example, treating a case of mycoplasma pneumonia with an antibiotic designed for a typical bacterial pneumonia may yield a partial response, lending some strength to the misdiagnosis of a bacterial pneumonia. However, the mycoplasma may not resolve as a result of this treatment, and may show a "puzzling" recurrence or even an exacerbation in following weeks.

The reverse of this problem also occurs: A correct diagnosis is made and appropriate treatment is begun. If the patient shows no response to treatment after a reasonable amount of time, the physician erroneously may be led to believe that the diagnosis was incorrect. There are many reasons for lack of response to a medical treatment other than an incorrect diagnosis or an ineffective therapy. For example, a patient may simply fail to adhere to the medical regimen prescribed, or may take only a partial course of medication because of uncomfortable side effects. The resulting "lack of response" may convince the physician to consider an alternate diagnosis (which would, under such circumstances, be an error).

The remaining sections of this chapter focus primarily on making therapeutic decisions and prognostic judgments with the assumption that a correct diagnosis has been made. However, it is important to bear in mind that our views of the efficacies of many medical therapies evaluated in research studies are likely to be confounded by instances in which an incorrect diagnosis has been the starting point. In addition, estimates of efficacy depend on whether patient adherence with the regimen has been adequate—something that may be difficult if not impossible to determine with a comfortable degree of accuracy.

■LINKING TREATMENT DECISIONS WITH PROGNOSES

This chapter deals with both treatment decisions and prognoses because the two are connected in an essential way. What makes one medical treatment preferable over another? When there are options in the treatments available for a disease, how is a particular treatment selected? To a great extent, treatment decisions are made on the basis of prognoses associated with different medical options. Frequently, prognoses take the form of **life expectancies.** A cancer patient might ask, "What is my life expectancy if I undergo extensive chemotherapy after my surgery in contrast to my life expectancy if I refuse chemotherapy?" Prognoses may also take the form of **quality of life** associated with treatment options. An avid tennis player might ask, "Which course of treatment is more likely to get me back on my feet on the tennis court—arthroscopic surgery or total knee replacement?"

There is, in fact, no sense in discussing medical options without bringing in issues of prognosis. After all, the point of treatment is to achieve a goal; and prognosis is an estimate of the likelihood that the goal will be achieved, whether it is an extension of life expectancy, a particular quality of life, or both.

Like most medical information, prognostic information rarely is exact. Prognoses consist of probabilities that a particular outcome will occur. Consequently, when the cancer patient asks whether he will live longer if he opts for chemotherapy after surgery instead of surgery alone, the physician cannot provide a definitive "yes" or "no" answer. The physician's answer may be stated in terms of "more likely" or "less likely," and perhaps will contain some quantitative estimates of the probabilities in question, e.g., "For your particular cancer, you are about 20% more likely to survive for 5 years if you take the chemotherapy than if you do not."

Prognostic judgments are made on the basis of two major sources of medical information: (1) Existing studies of groups of people who have undergone a particular treatment and (2) specific information about the individual patient being treated, which might affect response to treatment. Information about the individual being treated is essential in order to tailor the findings from large-scale investigations more closely to the characteristics of the individual case. When there is an absence of scientific studies, when studies are very new, or when different studies yield conflicting results, expert physicians may participate in a kind of survey called a Delphi technique, which is an attempt to arrive at a consensus opinion about which course of medical action is best. While the opinions of experts can be extremely valuable, expert opinions are not the same kind of information as data obtained from scientific studies. Sometimes they are more useful because they reflect real-life clinical experience. And sometimes they represent a bias that pervades the subculture of physicians. Such was the unfortunate case when physicians continued to prescribe diethystilbestrol to prevent miscarriages because authorities in the obstetrics field "believed" in the drug—even though research had begun to reveal the fact that the drug produced serious teratogenic (deforming) effects in the fetus.

■TO TREAT OR NOT TO TREAT—WHEN THAT IS THE QUESTION

The mandate to ". . .do no harm" (an essential part of the Hippocratic Oath taken by physicians) is not always easy to follow. What constitutes harm? Depending on the vantage points of the physician and the patient, something that is "harmful" in one case may not be judged as "harmful" in another. Here is a critical door through which **subjective values** enter into treatment decisions.

Primary liver cancer continues to defy treatment. With or without chemotherapy, the life expectancy of a patient diagnosed with this condition rarely is more than months. The chemotherapies available for this cancer are heavy-hitting medicines often accompanied by unpleasant and debilitating side-effects. However, it is possible that the use of chemotherapy might achieve a brief extension of life for some patients.

Which is more harmful: treating the patient with a chemotherapy, which has a poor chance of extending life by even a few months while causing miserable side-effects, or withholding the therapy and letting nature take its course?

The answer to what is harmful often can be found in the patient's subjective values. While one patient might opt for heroic measures to sustain life, another might feel like a laboratory rat being subjected to yet another ordeal that is not worth 2 more months of a miserable existence. In spite of the fact that some patients are quite clear about their medical preferences, it is not necessarily easy for the physician to acquiesce to patient wishes. Some patients with terminal illnesses might prefer to avoid some if not most of the medical therapies available to achieve an extension of their lives. Knowing that there is no cure for their disease, they might opt for no treatment at all, or even for physician-assisted suicide in lieu of a regimen of therapies that might cause even more discomfort than they have endured already. Under such circumstances, how can the treating physician best serve the patient and remain true to the dictum to *do no harm?*

In Western medicine, there appears to be a bias on the part of many physicians to do something rather than nothing, even if doing something is unlikely to be of benefit to the patient (Jordan et al.,1994). The continuous availability of new therapies lends power to the bias to do something, because there appears always to be some new option that might work, even if it is still in early experimental stages. Cancer therapies, for example, are changing so rapidly that an on-line information base called ONCOSIN was developed to provide data on the newest treatment options, even before reports of some of these appear in the medical journals. With many treatment options available for many diseases, contemporary physicians tend to be biased toward treating patients even when the hope of cure is remote and little evidence exists that any other kind of benefit can be achieved.

Even in this era of high-tech medicine, there are times when no treatment may be the best treatment. A tear in the miniscus of the knee due to a skiing injury might resolve by itself, without the assistance of arthroscopic surgery. A woman with lobular carcinoma in situ might not require preventive bilateral mastectomy in order to avoid invasive cancer. On the other hand, a patient with multiple myeloma might survive 4 years rather than 4 months if treated with appropriate chemotherapy. And those 4 years might represent a good quality of life, including the opportunity to do some things a patient had hoped to do during his lifetime.

Ultimately, the question of whether to treat or not hinges on prognosis, as well as on subjective values.

■THE INEVITABILITY OF TRADE-OFFS

Are the possible benefits of hormone replacement therapy (HRT) for menopausal women worth the risks that appear to be associated with the therapy? A woman might present this dilemma to her physician: "I want HRT because I am fearful of bone loss and because I want to give myself optimal protection against heart disease, but I am also fearful of the increased risks of breast cancer and endometrial cancer that seem to go along with HRT. What should I do?" Research on bone loss, i.e., osteoporosis, suggests that women lose a significant percentage of bone density, perhaps 2 to 3% per year, in the years after menopause. Many older women sustain fractures, including debilitating hip fractures, which might be avoided if loss of bone density were minimized by HRT. There also is evidence to suggest that the female hormone estrogen confers some protection against heart disease. On the other hand, these possible benefits are countered by concerns about increased risk of endometrial cancer and, even more seriously, of breast cancer.

The question of whether a woman should receive HRT illustrates a dilemma in modern medicine. With many treatment possibilities have come many trade-offs that must be considered. Some of the questions that would need to be answered before an HRT treatment decision could be made might include: What is the patient's personal and family history of heart disease, breast cancer, and endometrial cancer? Does the patient show a frail or slight body build, which might make her prone to serious effects of bone loss? Which other symptoms, if any, is she experiencing (e.g., hot flashes, mood swings, vaginal discomfort) that might be interfering with the quality of her life and that might be relieved by HRT? In some way, the risks as well as the benefits of the treatment must be weighed in order to arrive at the best medical decision for the patient.

Trade-offs seem to be an unavoidable aspect of contemporary medical decisions. Very often, the most effective treatments also are the most risky, most invasive/uncomfortable, and most expensive. This is true also of diagnostic testing, in which the most accurate tests for a disease tend to be those that carry the greatest risk, discomfort, and cost.

While trade-offs characterize many diagnostic problems as well as many therapeutic problems, there is an essential difference in the way diagnostic trade-offs and therapeutic trade-offs affect patients: In many situations, as explained in detail in Chapter 4, a medical diagnosis most often is made using more than one test. In fact, the diagnostic process often begins with less invasive testing and moves to more invasive testing only when necessary, in the hope that the less invasive tests will yield sufficiently good information to make a diagnostic conclusion without going any further. There certainly are down-sides to this step-by-step work up for a medical problem, including the time it takes to arrive at a diagnosis. However, most diagnostic procedures are not what we would call "irrevocable." Treatment decisions are more likely to have irrevocable consequences: A man undergoes prostate surgery and becomes impotent as a result; a woman undergoes preventive bilateral mastectomy because biopsy findings suggest that she is at extremely high risk for invasive cancer; a premenopausal woman has a complete hysterectomy to treat excessive menstrual bleeding and is no longer able to bear children. Nonsurgical treatment decisions can also have irreversible consequences: A woman is not provided HRT and suffers severe osteoporosis and hip fracture; a middle-aged man begins aspirin therapy to prevent heart disease and suffers a stroke as a result; a patient with nonactive tuberculosis complies with preventive therapy and dies from liver toxicity.

When medical decision making becomes too complex to be managed in "our heads," we can use informatics tools to help weigh the risks and benefits. Decision analysis is the primary tool that has been used for this purpose during the past two decades. It is described in detail later in this chapter.

Using Existing Studies to Make Treatment Decisions ....

■SINGLE REPORTS AND CASE STUDIES

There are times when reports of a single case can alter the course of a science. If a single patient with HIV disease achieved a cure, medical treatment of this virus would be revolutionized. However, most research on contemporary medical therapies is not so clear and unequivocal.

Consider two major disease categories of great concern to Western cultures: heart disease and cancer. Studies that attempt to investigate methods for preventing heart disease have been equivocal. Drug therapies designed to reduce cholesterol clearly do not benefit all patients, nor are they free of side effects. Investigation of aspirin to prevent myocardial infarction showed no difference in mortality from cardiovascular causes between a treatment and a control group. However, a statistically significant lowering of risk of heart attack was found in the aspirin group, but this finding was accompanied by a statistically significant increased risk of serious stroke (Steering Committee of the Physicians' Health Study Research Group, 1989). What is the best treatment for an already occluded coronary artery: angioplasty that might need to be repeated every 6 months, or bypass surgery? If bypass is selected, should the procedure be performed using the traditional open-chest surgery or the very new laparoscopic technique? Studies on cancer prevention as well as treatment are also replete with controversy. For many types of cancer, there are ongoing clinical trials aimed at determining which kind of adjuvant therapy, i.e., which combinations of chemo or chemo plus radiation yield the longest life expectancy. While progress is being made, there remains a wide range of patient responses to various regimens: a heavy-hitting regimen that might buy one patient another 5 years of life might result in a serious secondary infection in another.

Attempting to make a medical decision on the basis of individual studies can be very difficult, since results tend to vary from study to study. And within each study, responses to treatments vary from patient to patient. Results typically are reported as some form of average: an average life expectancy, a relative risk calculated on average responses to treatments, an average improvement in quality of life. And "averages" are typically accompanied by measurements of "error," including error bands in data charts and reports of standard deviations. These measurements of error are vastly important because they provide information about the extent to which individual patients have responded differently from the average calculated on their group. When error bands are large, using the results to make judgments about individual patients is risky. On the other hand, some studies report only small error bands and, therefore, may be more useful in clinical practice. For example, in an article published in *The Lancet* on the efficacy of adjuvant therapies for women with early stage breast cancer, the researchers reported that the effects of tamoxifen were so similar across patients that error bars could not even be printed on the graphs: They were smaller than the dots and squares used to plot the average numbers of recurrences and deaths over time! (See p. 6, Early Breast Cancer Trialists' Collaborative Group, 1992.)

What this means is that it is difficult to read a study performed on groups of patients and to decide to what extent the results apply to any individual patient who requires treatment for the disease investigated in the article. Then consider reading several or many articles on the same topic. Not only are there differences among patients in each article, but also there are typically differences in the findings across studies.

The crux of the problem is this: Except in very unusual circumstances, people typically do not respond in identical ways to an identical therapy. Because study after study has shown that individual differences occur in responses to medical treatments, researchers have moved increasingly to large sample studies instead of studies of small samples or single cases. The rationale is that if studies enroll large enough numbers of patients, the individual differences will somehow balance out— meaning that there will be as many poor responders as excellent responders, and that the overall effect of this balance will give a meaningful "average" result that the reader can accept as the best estimate of a therapy's efficacy. While there certainly are problems with best estimates, having an estimate usually is preferable to having no estimate at all.

As the information explosion continues, the medical literature expands with so many studies on some topics that it becomes impossible for the human brain to make enough sense of it to arrive at a meaningful conclusion to a question that might be as straightforward as, "Is chemotherapy alone or chemotherapy plus radiation the best choice for my patient with Stage II breast cancer?"

One of the techniques that has been developed to assist readers to integrate the results of many studies is called **meta-analysis** which is, in a sense, studying studies.

■SUMMARY DATA IN THE FORM OF META-ANALYSIS

Meta-analysis can be viewed as both a help and a hindrance in making treatment decisions. Since it is one way of "summarizing" the findings on a given topic, it can reduce the confusion of multiple and often contradictory investigations to a few quantitative estimates. On the other hand, it moves the consumer of research even further away from the picture of the individual patient: Individual differences among patients are no longer visible in meta-analyses because the individual differ-ences of concern in these analyses are **differences across studies.**

In order to evaluate the usefulness of meta-analysis in making treatment decisions, it is helpful to understand how such "secondary" analyses are done, as well as the cautions that are associated with each step along the way. Meta-analyses in medicine, as in any other field, proceed according to the following steps:

Step 1

After a topic is selected, an exhaustive search of the literature is conducted to identify all relevant investigations.

Caution: Even the best search strategies are unlikely to turn up all relevant investigations. There are at least two reasons for this limitation: First, even highly respected computerized litera-ture retrieval systems, such as MEDLINE, cannot be expected to contain all relevant literature. For example, MEDLINE does not provide full texts of foreign language (i.e., non-English) publications, nor does it incorporate doctoral dissertations or many conference presentations. Consequently, some state-of-the-art information can escape retrieval. Second, as in many fields, the medical literature suffers from a bias toward publish-ing studies that report statistically significant results. This means that studies which show statistically significant effects will predominate over studies that do not, simply because the latter are less likely to be published regardless of the quality of the investigation.

Step 2

Criteria are set for inclusion and exclusion of studies from the meta-analysis. Criteria may involve the adequacy of studies based on sample sizes, study designs, sites of investigations, etc. This step may also include the development of a system for differentially weighting studies that are considered to be "stronger" than others.

Caution: This a an extremely subjective aspect of the meta-analysis. Some researchers will elect to weight well-designed studies more highly than poorly designed studies. The weights that are assigned are arbitrary. Some researchers will weight large sample studies more highly than small sample studies, again according to an arbitrarily devised weighting system. Yet other researchers will decide to exclude completely poorly designed or small sample studies from their meta-analysis. There are no definitive guidelines for weighting systems or inclusion/exclusion criteria. Consequently, the reader must be sure that the meta-analysis contains a clear description of how such systems and criteria were applied—and must draw intelligent conclusions about the ways in which these systems and criteria might bias the results of the meta-analysis.

Step 3

Summary data are extracted from each of the studies selected for inclusion in the meta-analysis. What is looked for at this stage are "effect sizes," i.e., the impact of a therapy in terms of life extension, quality of life, and relative risk.

Caution: An individual study might show a large difference between a treatment and a control group, or across several treatment groups, but the difference might not be statistically significant. What is extracted from each study, for the purposes of meta-analysis, is the size of the difference between or among groups, not the level of statistical significance. So, why does statistical significance matter? Remember, statistical significance is a check on the likelihood that what has been found in a study sample is reflective of a broader population. Lack of statistical significance, in the presence of a large difference in group responses to treatment, may mean that the sample sizes in the study are too small to yield reliable results, or that individual differences within groups (i.e., standard deviations) are so large that they overshadow the differences found between groups (i.e., group averages). Thinking back to Step 2, some researchers will exclude studies that do not reach statistical significance from their meta-analysis. The downside to this is that some studies do not reach statistical significance because there really is no difference between groups of patients subjected to different therapeutic regimens! There is no easy resolution to this dilemma, except to be aware of how studies get selected for inclusion and the biases which might result from particular selection criteria.

Step 4

Statistical analyses are conducted on the data extracted in Step 3. These analyses yield summary numbers that indicate the overall efficacy of a treatment across all investigations that have been included, as well as an indication of variability or error across investigations.

Caution: Remember, in interpreting the results of the meta-analysis that this technique is a study of studies. It is vulnerable to all the cautions raised under Steps 1 through 3 above. Do not assume that the results of such an analysis can be applied directly to an individual patient. Such an assumption involves what is known as the "ecological fallacy." This means that you cannot go from one unit of analysis, i.e., the study as "subject" of research, to another unit of analysis, i.e., the individual patient, without making an unfounded leap. The leap is this: Once you have gotten to the level of meta-analysis, you have lost sight of individual differences among people, because the individual differences calculated in meta-analyses are differences among studies. And the studies included in meta-analyses may be so different from each other, that the task amounts to comparing apples with oranges. It is very hard to see the applications to an individual case from the meta level of meta-analysis.

An example of the use of meta-analysis might help to clarify some of the above points. The National Centers for Disease Control commissioned a meta-analysis on the efficacy of bacillus-Calmette-Guérin (BCG) vaccine for the prevention of tuberculosis (Colditz et al., 1994). The meta-analysis included studies from many countries using different strains of the BCG vaccine. Individual investigations in the meta-analysis included studies in which zero efficacy was associated with BCG as well as studies that reported an efficacy of 100% in preventing active tuberculosis. Studies varied greatly in design, ranging from loose correlational studies to more careful experimental and quasi-experimental designs. No studies were excluded, and no weighting criteria were applied. However, results were compiled for all studies together as well as separately for experimental versus nonexperimental studies. Overall, the meta-analysis concluded that BCG is approximately 50% effective in preventing TB.

How should this summary result be used in making treatment decisions for individual patients? Should BCG vaccine be given to everyone in the belief that it will prevent TB 50% of the time? Should it be given to health care workers in U.S. hospitals to reduce the incidence of active TB? And, finally, should an individual physician in the United States vaccinate an individual patient with BCG?

Hopefully, it is obvious from the above example that meta-analyses can take us so far afield from individual cases that they can be virtually useless in making treatment decisions. For any individual, BCG might be completely ineffective or completely effective, or anything in between.

In addition, meta-analyses are not built to weigh trade-offs inherent in treatment decisions. In the BCG example, the meta-analysis could not factor in the critical down side of the vaccine: the fact that once individuals are inoculated, they will show a positive tuberculin skin test regardless of whether they have become infected with the disease. This means that there will be no way to determine whether or not they have, in fact, become infected with the tubercle bacillus because the test has been invalidated by the vaccine. Consequently, therapy to prevent active, contagious disease typically is not given to individuals who have been inoculated with BCG, except under very specific circumstances. In other words, the inevitability of trade-offs warrants techniques that can consider both the pros and cons of a course of medical action—something meta-analysis is not built to do.

Perhaps one of the best uses of meta-analysis is not as a clinical decision tool, but rather as a way to understand the amount of agreement or disagreement currently existing on a controversial topic. If viewed from this perspective, it can be of substantial value.

■DECISION ANALYSIS

Like meta-analysis, decision analysis typically uses existing data to arrive at conclusions about which course of medical action is preferred. However, in contrast to meta-analysis, decision analysis is built specifically to handle the trade-offs inherent in medical practice. Consequently, decision analysis has become the premier informatics tool for making therapeutic decisions that involve complex trade-offs.

The steps and cautions associated with decision analysis can be thought out in a manner similar to that used for meta-analysis above. A more extensive discussion of the method is presented in the following section, Constructing and Interpreting Decision Models.

Step 1

Build a decision "tree." This tree must contain the relevant medical choices under consideration, for example, three approaches to the treatment of hypertension. For each medical choice, every possible result must also be included in the tree. Typically, decision trees contain "branches" that show good results and poor results, side effects and no side effects. Following the example of hypertension, these branches might include control of hypertension and lack of control, as well as such side effects as dizziness and impotence.

A "generic" decision tree for only two options, which might help in conceptualizing this phase of the process, is shown in Figure 6a.

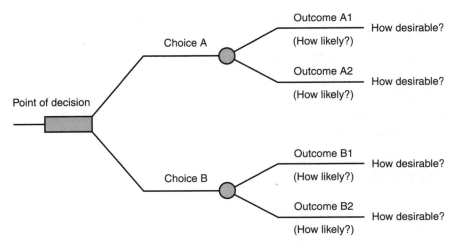

Figure 6a Generic decision tree.

Caution: In developing a decision tree, it is crucial to include all possible outcomes, even if the likelihood of occurrence is extremely small. In other words, a decision tree should exhaust all possibilities that can result from each course of action under consideration. Without a truly complete model, all further steps can be deceiving.

Step 2

For each "effect" associated with each branch of a decision tree, a probability estimate must be assigned. Using existing research, the question to be answered, is: How likely is this to occur? Using the "generic" tree shown in Figure 6a, the questions to be answered are: How likely is it that the disease will persist—or resolve— if treated? How likely is the treatment to produce side effects? How likely is it that the disease will persist—or resolve—if untreated? How likely is it for side effects to be associated with no treatment? (This last question might seem absurd. However, research has shown that in blinded studies, placebo groups sometimes report side effects in spite of the absence of treatment. This probability can serve as a baseline for the everyday discomforts that might be mistakenly factored into undesirable treatment effects.)

Caution: Think about where the probabilities for each branch of a decision tree come from. The answer usually is existing research. How does the decision analyst decide which study or studies to use to obtain these probabilities? And, if existing research shows equivocal results, has the decision model been developed with a bias toward one perspective rather than another? The example of decision analysis used to decide whether to administer or withhold preventive therapy for tuberculosis hinged on a battle over probability estimates for more than a decade. This example is discussed in detail below.

Step 3

In addition to assigning probabilities to each branch in a decision tree, a value must be assigned to each endpoint. An endpoint is an ultimate outcome reached after following from left to right, all the effects that have occurred after selecting a course of action. For example, a value will be assigned to the topmost path in the generic decision tree in Figure 6a. This path consists of treating the patient, the patient's disease resolving, but side effects having occurred as a consequence of treatment. How good is this path in contrast to other paths in the same tree? Is it as good as having the disease resolve without treatment and without side effects? Some way must be found to assign values to each of the endpoints.

Caution: Assigning values to endpoints in a decision model is probably the most subjective aspect of decision analysis. Some treatments are designed to extend life, so researchers might use life expectancies as endpoints. But life expectancies alone often are insufficient. For example, is it as good to survive an additional 5 years with debilitating side effects as it is to survive an additional 5 years without side effects? To address this kind of issue, many decision analysts incorporate quality of life into their decision models. But how is this done? And, whose perceptions of quality of life are used? Frequently, researchers use what is known as Quality Adjusted Life Years (QUALYs) to incorporate both life expectancies and life quality. However, the decision model cannot be truly reflective of the choices confronting a specific patient unless that patient's values are reflected in the decision tree. All too often, the quality-of-life adjustments that are made in decision models are physicians' best estimates of what patients' values might be, rather than values actually obtained from discussions with individual patients.

Step 4

Analyzing the decision tree. After Steps 1 through 3 have been carried out, the decision tree can be analyzed. The analysis proceeds from right to left (the reverse of how the tree was developed), in a mathematical process known as "averaging out and folding back." First, utility values are multiplied against the probabilities of the branches immediately to their left. Then the products are multiplied against the probabilities contained in the next branches, until all probabilities have been used. To learn more about this process, which is not nearly as complicated as it sounds, see the extended section on Constructing and Interpreting Decision Models. Finally, a number is obtained for each course of medical action considered in the decision tree. In the simple example used in this section and shown in Figure 6a, a number would be obtained for the choice "Treat" as well as for the choice "Don't Treat." Because decision models usually are constructed to determine which course of action maximizes both life expectancy and life quality, the choice with the highest number "wins." (If cost were used as an endpoint, then the choice with the lowest number would "win.")

Caution: In evaluating the results of a decision analysis, there are no guidelines to inform us as to what is a meaningful difference between or among courses of action. If the "Treat" branch winds up with a Quality Adjusted Life Years score of 5.5 years, and the "Don't Treat" branch winds up with a score of 5.4 years, is that difference sufficient to recommend treatment? Under what circumstances is one tenth of a year of life enough to justify one course of action over others? And what about weeks, days, or even hours of life, as is sometimes the case? There are no tests of statistical significance to assist in determining what constitutes a meaningful difference once the decision tree is analyzed. Consequently, two clinicians looking at the same decision analysis results might form completely different conclusions.

While it is clear that decision analysis is vulnerable at many points, particularly the point at which values are assigned to endpoints on the tree, this element of subjectivity can be seen as a strength of the technique rather than a weakness. Being able to tailor a decision to the values of a specific individual or to a particular population enables the health care provider to go beyond the objective but impersonal results of scientific studies and to inject a "human element" into medical choices.

Decision analysis made its major debut in the medical literature in the argument about whether to prescribe isoniazid preventive therapy for what were termed low-risk tuberculin reactors. Essentially, the argument centered on two points: First, when someone is found to have a positive TB skin test, without a clear idea of how or when the initial infection occurred, it is virtually impossible to estimate their risk of developing active, contagious disease. These individuals are termed low-risk reactors because they are unlikely to have contacted the TB bacillus recently and, therefore, are probably at a relatively low risk for developing active disease. (Recall that TB is a two-stage process. Only about 10% of individuals infected with TB who are not immune-compromised go on to develop active, contagious disease during their lifetimes. For the remaining vast majority, the only consequence of having contacted the organism is a positive skin test.) Second, isoniazid preventive therapy has been shown to be toxic to the liver in a small percentage of patients, a risk that increases with age. Stated in decision analysis terms, the trade-off in question is whether it is preferable to give isoniazid preventive therapy to low-risk reactors aged 35 and older, knowing that these individuals face a risk of liver toxicity, or to withhold preventive therapy knowing that these individuals may develop active, contagious disease.

To see how decision analysis was used to shed light on the argument about preventive therapy for TB, read the following section.

Constructing and Interpreting Decision Models.........................

Since the mid-1970s the American Thoracic Society in conjunction with the Centers for Disease Control recommended that anyone younger than 35 years who has a positive tuberculin skin test and no specific contraindications should receive preventive therapy with isoniazid. The purpose of this medical regimen is to prevent initial infection with the tubercle bacillus from becoming active, contagious disease. In 1981, a group of researchers used decision analysis to question this recommendation, and concluded that the risk of isoniazid-related hepatitis did not outweigh the benefit of TB prevention (Taylor et al., 1981). Five years later, another group of researchers reexamined this issue, also using decision analysis, and concluded that the benefits of isoniazid preventive therapy do outweigh its risks throughout a 10- to 80-year lifespan (Rose et al., 1986). These conflicting decision analyses reopened the great debate over isoniazid preventive therapy for TB. They also showcased a method relatively new to clinical medicine: decision analysis.

A number of other studies followed in the path of these conflicting analyses, investigating such issues as the use of isoniazid in nursing homes and the cost-effectiveness of longer versus shorter term therapy. In 1988, a decision analysis designed to resolve the isoniazid dilemma reported yet another "take" on the problem: that the decision was too close to call one way or the other. In fact, this study was titled, *Isoniazid for the Tuberculin Reactor: Take It or Leave It* (Tsevat et al., 1988). In an editorial in the same journal, the Director of Tuberculosis Control for the Centers for Disease Control raised numerous criticisms of the analysis, which focused primarily on the probabilities that were used in the decision model (Snider, 1988).

The arguments over isoniazid preventive therapy provide classic examples of decision analysis used to make treatment choices and also highlight some of the cautions regarding decision analysis that were discussed in the previous section of this chapter. While researchers were in close agreement on the structure of the decision tree to be used in the analysis, battles were waged over the choice of probability estimates, outcome values, and what constitutes a "meaningful" difference rather than a "toss-up."

To provide a detailed illustration of the steps and pitfalls involved in performing a decision analysis on a relatively complex treatment problem, the following sections describe the process that culminated in a 1991 article that revisited the isoniazid dilemma yet again (Jordan et al., 1991).

■DEVELOPING A DECISION TREE

Figure 6b shows the decision tree for outcomes that result from withholding or prescribing isoniazid (INH) preventive therapy for an individual with a positive tuberculin skin test.

Beginning with the bottom of the decision tree and reading from left to right, a No INH choice can result either in the patient never getting active TB or getting active TB. If the patient develops active TB, he or she would be treated with an appropriate treatment regimen, usually a combination of isoniazid, rifampin, and pyrazinamide. The patient may or may not develop hepatotoxicity (liver disease) from treatment of active TB. Without hepatotoxicity, the patient will either survive TB or die from it. With hepatotoxicity, the patient will either survive this liver disease or not. If the patient survives hepatotoxicity, it remains to be seen whether he or she will survive TB or die from it. These paths take us to the end of the No INH branches of the tree.

The INH choice repeats many of the same contingencies, but is more complicated because it begins with the immediate possibilities that the patient will or will not develop hepatotoxic-

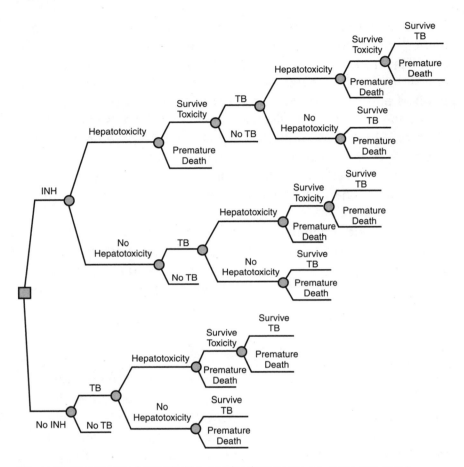

Figure 6b Decision tree for isoniazid preventive therapy. [Source: Jordan et al., 1991.]

ity from the preventive therapy. If there is no hepatotoxicity from the preventive therapy, the rest of the contingencies are identical to those shown in the No INH choice. If there is hepatotoxicity from INH preventive therapy, one additional branching is needed to show whether the patient survives this hepatotoxicity or dies from it.

One of the pitfalls which can occur in constructing this decision model is the failure to consider that individuals who develop active TB, whether or not they have received INH preventive therapy, will be treated with an INH-containing regimen, which is also hepatotoxic. Other studies did not include this additional branch in their decision models.

■DERIVING PROBABILITY ESTIMATES

Decision analysts look to existing literature to obtain estimates of the likelihoods that each of the contingencies represented in their trees will occur. Previous studies drew criticisms for using estimates that were either too high or too low. The position taken by the researchers who published this decision analysis was that the numbers confusion arose in part because previous estimates grouped all patients together, failing to consider that existing literature showed that risks appear to differ according to the patient's gender and ethnicity.

Clearly, one of the pitfalls in selecting probabilities for a decision model is a failure to consider closely the characteristics of the sample from which probabilities were derived. Does it make good scientific sense to group all patients together? Or are some patients at greater or lesser risk than others?

In the INH decision model shown in Table 6a, the likelihood of dying from hepatotoxicity appeared to vary widely with ethnicity and gender. From Table 6a, it is clear that the risk of dying reported in existing literature (Kopanoff et al., 1978) was substantially higher for blacks, particularly for black women. Consequently, decision models that used overall averages or estimates for whites when the decision in question would affect blacks as well could have produced deceptive results.

TABLE 6a PROBABILITIES OF DYING FROM INH-RELATED HEPATOTOXICITY

	Female	Male
Black	12.5%	5.9%
White	2.6%	2.9%

■ASSIGNING VALUES TO ENDPOINTS

In this decision model, assigning values can be quite tricky. First, what is being valued? For some researchers, the focus might appear to be life and death. For others, it might appear to be impacted on quality of life from developing a contagious disease or not.

How would quantitative "scores" be assigned to these values? If the decision were as simple as life or death, then life could be assigned a 1 and death a zero. If quality of life were also being considered, then more fine-tuning could be required: For example, surviving without ever having active TB might get a score of 1, while surviving after having suffered through active disease might be less than 1, but not as bad as a score of zero (death). How much should be subtracted from a score of 1 to "adjust" for the negative experience of disease?

These questions illustrate some of the pitfalls involved in assigning values to endpoints. When patients were asked about how bad it would be to have active TB, even though they would survive, they responded in very different ways. Patients who had young children at home, and feared transmission to their families, scored active TB very low. Other patients, particularly those who had other serious medical problems such as heart disease, tended to place a high value on life even when survival involved having gone through active TB. Another pitfall in the assignment of values is to view all deaths as zero. This is because a patient who dies from INH preventive therapy typically dies within 12 to 18 weeks after beginning treatment. On the other hand, patients who die from active TB might not develop the active disease for another 10 to 20 years. Thus, someone who gets TB and dies from it is unlikely to die as early as someone who dies from INH preventive therapy. Consequently, all deaths in this decision model do not merit the same score of zero!

In order to avoid these pitfalls, the model under discussion used life expectancies initially as endpoints in the decision model. Consequently, dying from INH preventive therapy received a score of 15 weeks (the midpoint of 12–18 weeks), and dying from active TB received a score of 13 to 40 years, depending on the ethnicity, gender, and age of the patient at diagnosis of infection. While this system of assigned values addressed the pitfall of equating very early deaths with much later deaths, it did not assist in making quality-of-life adjustments for developing active disease. Because this seemed to be such a personal, individualized matter for patients who were interviewed, it was thought best to leave Quality Adjusted Life Years to be done for individual cases who would work through the decision with their physicians.

■**ANALYZING AND INTERPRETING THE DECISION MODEL**

Remember that this decision problem started as a challenge to a policy recommended for most Americans by the American Thoracic Society and the Centers for Disease Control. This means that the treatment problem was conceptualized first as an issue of public policy. In order to address public policy, the decision model published by Jordan et al. (1991) provided analyses for groups of people rather than for individual cases. This means that individual values could not be incorporated in the analyses, but that the analyses were performed separately by age, ethnicity, and gender. (Previous decision analyses had considered only age in their models.)

Results of the 1991 study favored prescribing INH preventive therapy for all 20-year olds, all 35-year olds except black women, and no 50-year olds. The findings suggested that ethnicity and gender as well as age were needed in decision analyses done on this topic.

However, consider this: In the subgroups for whom INH preventive therapy was preferred, it was selected because of a life expectancy benefit of only 3 to 19 days. Is this a meaningful difference? Or is this result also merely a "toss-up?"

At this point, it is difficult to know what constitutes a "meaningful" difference. In fact, a highly respected group of researchers had devoted a considerable amount of thought to the problem of differences in decision analysis (Kassirer et al., 1987), and were unable to offer a solution. Consequently, one of the final pitfalls in decision analysis lies in interpreting the results. What should be said about the 3- to 19-day benefit in life expectancy? Over many thousands, or hundreds of thousands of people infected with TB, these days add up to many, many years. On the other hand, to an individual patient, this "benefit" might not seem to be much of a benefit at all.

If the analysis part of decision analysis still seems elusive, that is because the actual mathematics have not been shown for this example. There are excellent computer programs that perform the mathematics, as well as textbooks that provide examples of gradually increasing difficulty in which the models are solved "by hand." Recommendations for further reading provided at the end of this chapter will be of great use in pursuing decision analysis in depth.

■GOING EVEN FURTHER

While the teaching example used in this section is complex, several points of decision analysis were omitted from the discussion because they are somewhat beyond the grasp of the first-time reader. However, it is important to know that there are some additional decision analysis techniques that will be found in some research, and that an understanding of these techniques can be obtained from reading texts devoted to decision analysis. Most importantly, these techniques are:

Sensitivity Anaysis

Sensitivity analysis is a powerful procedure that permits the researcher to explore the impact of different probabilities and utility values on the result of the decision analysis. This is especially useful when the literature contains wide-ranging estimates of probabilities, and when it is unclear which is the most correct. The technique is called "sensitivity analysis" because it enables the researcher to investigate how "sensitive" the results of the analysis are to variations in one or more estimates. The ultimate question becomes: Does my result (choice of therapy) change if I use a different estimate for one or more branches in my model? Sensitivity analyses can also be used to evaluate the impact of different values on the outcome of the analysis.

Markov Chains

Markov chains enable the researcher to incorporate a time element in the decision model in a very specific manner. This is useful when a researcher wants to explore the impact of competing therapies over specific time frames. For example, decision models dealing with competing therapies for cancer might need to incorporate yearly points at which the likelihoods of recurrences, continued remissions, and deaths are evaluated before reentering the tree.

Making and Using Prognostic Judgments

In the decision model above, when we decided to use an estimate of 15 weeks survival for individuals who develop INH-toxicity, we were making a **prognostic judgment.** To be even more precise, the literature suggests a survival range of 12 to 18 weeks. This information was used in the decision model as an endpoint, a "value" in the tree. Prognostic judgments are used in decision analysis because, as noted early in this chapter, selecting a treatment without paying attention to prognosis makes no sense. However, prognostic judgments are used in many other ways besides formal decision models. When decisions are simple enough to be made without the need for complex decision tools, knowing the prognoses associated with competing therapies may be sufficient to make a choice.

■UNDERSTANDING THE MEANING OF PROGNOSIS

The first important question a patient who is experiencing symptoms typically asks the physician is, "What's wrong with me?" or, alternatively, "What [disease] do I have?"

The second important question usually has something to do with treatment, "What are my options?" or "Do I have to have surgery?"

The third question is typically the one that is most difficult for both patient and physician to handle, particularly in the case of a life-threatening condition. Every physician hears it: "How long do I have?" The meaning is clear. The patient is asking for a time frame, how much longer he or she will live. If the disease is not life-threatening, the third question may take many other forms, usually having to do with quality of life. Some examples include: "Will I be able to have children?" "Will this affect my ability to have sex?" "How long before I can ski again?" "Will I continue to have this pain?" "Can I still drive a car?" All these questions, ranging from how long the patient will live to whether driving will continue to be possible are questions requiring prognostic judgments. In some instances, a prognosis will be relatively straightforward. For example, a woman with uterine tumors requiring a hysterectomy will not be able to conceive children. In other instances, a prognosis will be filled with uncertainty. For example, a woman with Stage II breast cancer asks whether her cancer will kill her and if it will, then when? To provide a prognostic judgment for this patient requires the physician to be familiar with studies of patients as much like his patient as possible, especially insofar as stage of disease, type of tumor, and responsiveness to treatments are concerned.

It is probably helpful to consider separately prognoses for chronic diseases with protracted clinical courses, and prognoses for acute, life-threatening diseases. At the present stage of medical knowledge, osteoarthritis is considered a chronic disease, while some (but not all) cancers are acutely life-threatening. To clarify this last point, consider prostate cancer and non-HIV Kaposi's sarcoma. Both these cancers tend to progress slowly, and very often are not the cause of death for the patients. On the other hand, ovarian cancer, advanced colon and breast cancers, and primary liver cancer are life-threatening diseases. Consequently, all cancers do not necessarily belong in the same category of disease when considering prognostic judgments.

When a patient newly diagnosed with osteoarthritis asks for a prognosis, the prognosis for this chronic disease might be something like this: "Your osteoarthritis is severe enough right now to interfere with many of your day-to-day activities. It's causing you chronic pain and has already produced some disfiguring of the joints of your fingers and toes. This kind of arthritis tends to respond to anti-inflammatory medications. We will try you on a course of a nonsteroidal anti-inflammatory medication, and if it causes you gastrointestinal upset, we have many other medications we can try. Medical therapy will not reverse the damage your arthritis has already done to your joints, but it can slow down the degenerative disease process and ease your arthritic pain. You will probably continue to have difficulty with some of the things you have enjoyed doing in the past, such as playing the piano and sketching. On the other hand, activities that require you to move your joints might help relieve some of the stiffness you are experiencing." This somewhat long-winded, qualitative prognosis is the physician's judgment that the patient has a chronic disease with a long-term clinical course that can be assisted by medical therapy. There is no concern about altered life expectancy, and no pressing need to be extremely precise about a time frame. The patient simply will have osteoarthritis for the rest of his/her life, and the progression of damage to his/her joints most likely will be slowed down by appropriate medical treatment.

Qualitative judgments, such as the above, tend to be unsatisfactory in acutely life-threatening situations. A woman who has just undergone breast surgery for a malignant tumor that has been categorized as Stage II, estrogen-receptor negative, node-positive disease, will be likely to ask questions requiring quantitative information. Her prognosis might be stated in terms such as these: "Recent studies of women with Stage II breast cancer show that adjuvant therapy after surgery significantly impacts on survival. Overall, women who have some form of adjuvant therapy do about 30% better on a per-year survival basis than women who refuse further treatment after their surgery. Your node-positive status means that you have some spread of disease, so adjuvant therapy is particularly important. And because your tumor was estrogen-receptor positive, you are more likely to benefit from tamoxifen therapy than from the traditional chemotherapy regimens. With this therapy, your chance of surviving for 5 years is about 70%, and for 10 years about 50%. Of course these numbers are averages calculated on many women, and the nature of averages is that many women do far better than these figures, while others do not do as well."

The similarities and differences in prognostic information given for the two different kinds of diseases are summarized in Table 6b.

This section has provided a schematic view of two categories of diseases, which have been simplified for the sake of illustration. However, it is important to understand that many diseases straddle both categories. Chronic obstructive pulmonary disease (COPD), for example, is a long-term, chronic disease that is also a cause of death in some cases. On the other hand, there are acute conditions, such as the common cold or a painful sprained ankle, that are not life threatening for the vast majority of people. Consequently, prognoses for some diseases may contain elements of both chronic/long-term and acutely life-threatening conditions, while prognoses for others

TABLE 6b   NATURE OF PROGNOSTIC INFORMATION BY DISEASE CATEGORY

	Chronic Disease	Life-Threatening Disease
Kind of information	Usually qualitative	Usually quantitative
Link to treatment	Yes, but often a step-by-step process with focus on patient preference and response over time	Yes, often with comparative data on competing therapies
Use of Mathematical Models of Prognosis	Not usually necessary	Yes, often necessary
Use of Decision Models	Yes, if there are complex therapeutic trade-offs and quantitative data	Yes, if there are complex therapeutic trade-offs

such as the common cold might be on the "take two aspirin and call me in the morning" level.

■REVIEWING SOME COMMON PROGNOSTIC MODELS

Prognostic models are mathematical devices that have been developed from research studies in order to provide guidance about what to expect in the clinical course of a disease. As discussed above, these models are most often used when diseases are considered to be very serious/life-threatening, as well as when varying characteristics of the patient, the disease, or its treatment appear to impact on remission, recurrence, or life expectancy. Consequently, most prognostic models provide mathematically derived estimates of expected time to recurrence of disease and/or estimates of life expectancies.

This section focuses on three commonly encountered prognostic models: life tables, Kaplan-Meier analysis, and Cox regression. The purpose of examining these methods is not to teach sophisticated mathematical calculations but rather to impart an understanding of how medical information from these analyses can be interpreted as well as what the most glaring shortcomings are for each of them.

Recent versions of the Statistical Programs for the Social Sciences (SPSS) computer software contain a section titled "Survival Analysis." Life tables, Kaplan-Meier analysis, and Cox regression are found under this category. Consequently, it is obvious that these three widely used techniques focus on prognostic information in the form of life expectancies.

Life Tables

This statistical procedure yields actuarial tables, used to examine the distribution of times between two events, when the second event (usually mortality) has not necessarily occurred. Three questions come to mind immediately: What are actuarial tables? What is this distribution of times between two events? And, how can the analysis be performed if the second event has not necessarily occurred?

First, actuarial tables are organized data, usually presented in tabular form but also presented graphically, which provide information about life expectancy. The "fixed interval" most commonly used is the year. However, while the yearly interval is a conventional way of organizing data, other time intervals are also acceptable.

Why are life insurance rates higher for older individuals than for younger ones? The answer is that life insurance companies make use of actuarial data in the form of life tables to determine when an individual is expected to die. This leads into the second question about the distribution of two events. For the insurance company the two "events" are the age at which the individual is requesting life insurance and the age at which he or she is expected to die. Now, the meaning of the third puzzle becomes clear: The second event, which has not occurred as yet, is the death of the individual who is requesting insurance. Life tables provide estimates of when an individual is going to die, based primarily on the individual's present age.

Continuing with the life insurance example, consider the question of why life insurance premiums tend to be higher for men than for women. This is because life table analyses often are performed separately for subgroups of individuals whose demographic characteristics impact on life expectancy; and gender is one important characteristic. Table 6c is a life table for Americans calculated separately by age at birth, gender, and race (National Center for Health Statistics, 1994).

Where do the numbers in life tables come from? The general answer is large sample databases. More specifically, these data come from such sources as the U.S. Census, National Institutes of Health databases, National Center for Health Statistics, and data collected by insurance companies.

Life table data also may be presented in the form of curves. Using the data presented in Table 6c, Figure 6c shows the same information in a different graphic format.

One of the cautions to be heeded when using life tables to make prognostic judgments is that life tables often do not do an adequate job of providing life expectancy estimates for people with specific diseases. Most of the data found in life tables re-

TABLE 6c LIFE EXPECTANCY AT BIRTH, AT 65 YEARS, AND AT 75 YEARS, BY RACE AND SEX: SELECTED YEARS, 1900–1902 TO 1991

Age and Year	All Races			White		Black	
	Both Sexes	Male	Female	Male	Female	Male	Female
	Remaining life expectancy in years						
At birth							
1900–1902[1,2]	47.3	46.3	48.3	46.6	48.7	32.5[3]	33.5[3]
1950[2]	68.2	65.6	71.1	66.5	72.2	58.9	62.7
1960[2]	69.7	66.6	73.1	67.4	74.1	60.7	65.9
1970	70.8	67.1	74.7	68.0	75.6	60.0	68.3
1980	73.7	70.0	77.4	70.7	78.1	63.8	72.5
1991	75.5	72.0	78.9	72.9	79.6	64.6	73.8
At 65 years							
1900–1902[1,2]	11.9	11.5	12.2	11.5	12.2	10.4	11.4
1950[2]	13.9	12.8	15.0	12.8	15.1	12.9	14.9
1960[2]	14.3	12.8	15.8	12.9	15.9	12.7	15.1
1970	15.2	13.1	17.0	13.1	17.1	12.5	15.7
1980	16.4	14.1	18.3	14.2	18.4	13.0	16.8
1991	17.4	15.3	19.1	15.4	19.2	13.4	17.2
At 75 years							
1980	10.4	8.8	11.5	8.8	11.5	8.3	10.7
1991	11.1	9.5	12.1	9.5	12.1	8.7	11.2

(Data are based on the National Vital Statistics System.)
[1] Death registration area only. The death registration area increased from 10 States and the District of Columbia in 1900 to the coterminous United States in 1933.
[2] Includes deaths of nonresidents of the United States.
[3] Figure is for the Black and other races population.
Source: National Center for Health Statistics, Health, United States, 1993, Hyattsville, MD, Public Health Service, 1994, table 27.

flect the "general population" rather than populations with particular diseases at particular stages in their clinical course. Consequently, life tables tend to be more useful in determining what is known as normal life expectancies for people of different ages, genders, and ethnicities, rather than for people with specific, different medical conditions.

Kaplan-Meier Analysis

While this statistical procedure is similar to life table analysis, there are some notable differences.

First, Kaplan-Meier analysis typically yields curves rather than data tables. This form of survival analysis uses existing

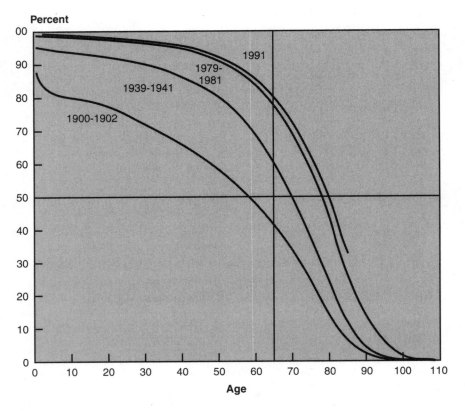

Figure 6c Graphic transformation of life table data.

data, often from individual research studies, to fit curves to patterns of data. In contrast to life tables (and curves based on life table data), Kaplan-Meier analyses frequently are performed on medically ill populations to determine the time from diagnosis of a disease to death.

In the Kaplan-Meier analysis, and in similar curve-fitting procedures, three phenomena are likely to take place in the research studies which provide the data:

1. During the time frame of the study, which typically is prospective and longitudinal, some of the patients die.

2. During the time frame of the study, some of the patients are likely to be lost to follow-up, meaning that no one really knows what has happened or what will happen to them.

3. At the point at which the study terminates, some of the patients may still be alive, so that the time of the second occurrence is unknown.

How is this third issue dealt with in the curve-fitting procedures? The answer is through extrapolation. Extrapolation is an educated guess about what would happen to people when they are no longer being monitored in the study. In other words, it is an estimate of when they will die, even though they have not died by the time the study terminates.

For an example of extrapolation in curve-fitting, see the curves in Figure 6d provided for women with early-stage breast cancer who have been treated with the adjuvant therapy tamoxifen.

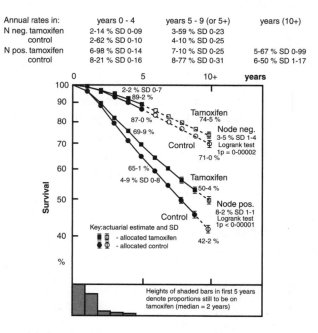

Figure 6d Actual and extrapolated life expectancies for women with early stage breast cancer. 3M—Mortality (all ages) in tamoxifen trials.

[Source: Early Breast Cancer Trialists' Collaborative Group, 1992. Reprinted with permission.]

The top two curves show percentage survival for women with node-negative cancers (i.e., no evidence of spread to lymph nodes) who have received either tamoxifen or no adjuvant therapy. Note that the squares and circles representing the two groups are darkened and connected by solid lines until the point in the figure denoting 5 years. After this point, the squares and circles are open and connected with a dotted line. Recall the curves of life table data presented earlier. The life table curves had no dotted or broken lines. In survival curves, dotted lines typically indicate areas in which extrapolation has been done, that is, areas for which actual data are no longer available. In this study, women on tamoxifen were not followed beyond 5 years, so the period from year 5 to year 10 is an estimate based on the kind of curve that was found to characterize the first 5 years of actual data. In the same example, the bottom two curves show percentage survival over time for node-positive patients (i.e., cancers that show lymph node involvement) who received either tamoxifen or no adjuvant therapy. Here, the actual data continue for 9 years. The dotted lines and open figures between years 9 and 10 indicate that extrapolations have been made.

The major caution regarding extrapolation is that it is not based on real data, and if women were followed for the full period of time shown in the figure, their actual survival might be quite different from the extrapolation. For example, some studies have suggested that if women have not died and have had no recurrences of their disease by 5 years after initial treatment for breast cancer, they have essentially achieved a cure. This would mean that the curves would not continue on their downward swing, but would flatten out.

Another caution to be heeded when using Kaplan-Meier and other such curve-fitting procedures to derive prognoses is the fact that even studies that begin with large samples of patients tend to lose patients very quickly if the disease is life-threatening. This means that the sample size on which some segments of the curve have been developed might be precariously small. Looking again at the tamoxifen example, notice that by year 5, only about 65% of the node-positive controls remain in the study. More than one-third of the women in this sample have already died from breast cancer. It is typical to see areas in such curves that contain either very few patients and/or a substantially reduced sample size. Curves based on small numbers can be quite unreliable, because occurrences in a few cases can impact drastically on the results: For example, 5 deaths out of 100 patients is only 5%, while 5 deaths out of a sample of 10 is 50%. Consequently, losses (deaths) incurred at the ends of curves where samples tend to be rather small can provide an exaggerated picture of the impact of the disease on life expectancy.

Cox Regression

This procedure is used to study the relation between the time it takes for an event to occur and a set of independent variables such as risk factors. As with the above techniques, the event of interest need not have occurred for all cases. By this time, it should be clear that survival analyses do not require that endpoints (death) be obtained for all cases in the study, because extrapolation can be used to make educated guesses about what is likely to occur. The major difference between Cox regression and the other two methods described above is that it permits the researcher to investigate the relation of other variables to life expectancy. Cox regression is performed when interest is directed not only at generating survival curves, but also in finding out whether additional variables can be used to improve prognostic judgments.

For example, in a study of life expectancies for patients with HIV disease, variables such as etiology and general health status might be important. Some researchers have suggested that patients who contract HIV disease through intravenous drug use have a shorter life expectancy than those whose route of contagion was sexual contact. General health status, including nutritional status, might also be predictive of life expectancy. In order to expand a survival analysis to include not only time to mortality but also possible contributing factors, a

Cox regression would be the procedure of choice. Results of the analysis would indicate the strength of the relation of contributing factors to life expectancy.

Cautions in using Cox regressions to make prognostic judgments include the cautions mentioned under Kaplan-Meier and other curve-fitting procedures, including the issue of extrapolation. In addition, while Cox regressions can provide valuable hints about variables which might be related to life expectancy, these relations cannot be interpreted as causes. As discussed in Chapter 3, causality can only hope to be inferred from strict experimental studies; Cox regressions are performed typically on nonexperimental data. This means that even if a variable such as nutritional status were strongly correlated with life expectancy in HIV disease, we cannot conclude with any degree of confidence that changing nutritional habits will improve a patient's prognosis.

■RECOGNIZING THE ELEMENTS OF UNCERTAINTY IN PROGNOSTIC JUDGMENTS

What we know about prognosis comes from how well or how poorly other individuals with the same disease have done. This means that making a prognosis about life expectancy for a patient who is still alive is based primarily on information about other patients. To what extent does information about other patients pertain to today's patient with HIV disease who is asking her physician, "How long do I have?" Existing data might be quite accurate; on the other hand, a cure for HIV disease might be discovered within the coming year, thus drastically changing this patient's prognosis. The emergence of antiretroviral therapies has drastically changed the prognosis for individuals with HIV disease from what it was before these new therapies became available.

Also, prognostic judgments are based on averages. As has been discussed earlier in this book, averages by definition mean that some people do better and some people do worse than this. Consequently, prognostic judgments based on large sample studies are inexact to the extent that they do not reflect individual differences, the variations among people that are relegated to statistics with names such as *standard deviation, error,* and *variance.* Using averages to make prognostic judgments can be helpful if both health care provider and patient clearly understand that averages are somewhat like rules that are meant to be broken. They are unhelpful if they are misinterpreted as absolute time frames because, seen as such, they may leave patients feeling either "cheated" out of the life expectancy promised by the survival analysis or, alternatively, deprived of the hope of possibly living longer than statistics say they will.

The Use of Receiver-Operating Characteristic Curves.........

This chapter began with a discussion of the importance of connecting treatment decisions to prognostic judgments and also noted that in order to make correct treatment decisions, it is necessary to begin with a correct diagnosis! Before concluding this chapter, it is important to revisit the relation between treatment decisions and accuracy of diagnosis.

In order to treat a patient for dandruff by prescribing a medicated shampoo, how sure does the physician need to be of the accuracy of the diagnosis? On the other hand, before performing a hysterectomy on a young woman suffering from severe abdominal pain and bleeding, how sure does the physician need to be that the source of the patient's symptoms is an irreversibly diseased uterus? Clearly, the levels of certainty required before medical action is taken differ dramatically in these two instances. The level of certainty required for action is called the **threshold.**

Receiver-operating characteristic (ROC) curves provide a method for identifying thresholds, based on the accuracy of diagnostic information. Figure 6e provides an illustration of a simple ROC curve used by Sainfort (1991) to teach the clinical applications of the technique.

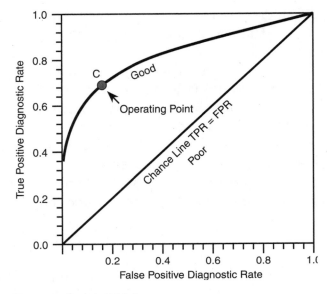

Figure 6e Sample ROC Curve.
[Source: Sainfort, 1991]

The diagonal line marked *poor* represents the point at which the number of true-positive diagnoses equals the number of false-positive diagnoses: In other words, the "corrects" are equal to the "errors" at this point. Such 50/50 odds are no better than flipping a coin to arrive at a diagnosis. Obviously, such a poor diagnostic capability would be acceptable only when a treatment is totally benign and inexpensive, such as suggesting the use of a medicated shampoo to treat dandruff.

On the other hand, test results that would be used to decide to perform a hysterectomy (such as endometrial biopsy and uterine ultrasound) must be excellent in order to convince physician and patient that the threshold for action has been reached. The curve marked *good* in Figure 6e shows more correct diagnoses and fewer errors: Its optimal threshold point or cutoff is marked "c." After this point, there are more false-positive diagnoses (e.g., not really a diseased uterus) which, in this case, do not outweigh the slight increases in correct diagnoses (true positives, e.g., a diseased uterus).

While ROC curves can be intimidating, they summarize diagnostic information in a visual manner, which can be more helpful to some people than simply knowing rates of true positives and true negatives. However, their greater strength resides in assisting the health care provider to "see" whether an acceptable threshold for action has been reached. Stated simply, when the course of medical action under consideration is drastic and irreversible, you will want a ROC curve that pulls to the upper left-hand corner of the graph, indicating that you are highly unlikely to be embarking on a treatment inappropriately. When the treatment under consideration is benign, a curve that is closer to the 50/50 line is less problematic.

Summary

We live in an era in which many treatment options may be available for a given disease. With treatment choices comes the dilemma of which treatment to choose. Selecting a treatment option is intimately linked to prognosis because prognosis is an estimate of how well or how poorly a patient is likely to respond. Selecting among treatment options typically involves weighing trade-offs: Options that tend to be most successful in resolving medical problems also tend to be the most risky, most uncomfortable, and most expensive. There are times when no treatment at all may be a reasonable course of action, particularly when available therapies are not very effective and are associated with highly undesirable side effects.

When the selection of a medical treatment is complicated by many options and many trade-offs, informatics "tools" can be used to assist patient and physician in making a treatment decision. Reports of single studies and summaries of studies in the form of meta-analyses can be helpful in developing an understanding of the state of clinical research in a particular area. However, in order to weigh trade-offs in a decision involving two or more therapeutic options, the tool of choice is decision analysis. Decision analysis is most useful when existing literature provides robust, unequivocal estimates of benefits and risks, and when both patients and health care providers are clear about the subjective values that enter into the decision.

Prognostic judgments made for chronic diseases that are not life threatening tend to rely on qualitative descriptions of what it will be like to live with a disease. In contrast, prognostic judgments made for life-threatening diseases will often rely on survival analyses that have been computed from large data sets or recent clinical research. These prognoses typically will be stated in quantitative terms, and will focus on life expectancies associated with different courses of medical action. Some common kinds of survival analysis include life tables, Kaplan-Meier analysis, and Cox regression.

Quantitative models of prognosis vary in their usefulness depending on the extent to which the patients who were studied are like the patient for whom a prognostic judgment is being made. Other factors that raise cautions about these models include the use of extrapolation beyond the point at which actual data are available, and losing so many research participants that parts of the model are based on very few participants. On the other hand, good prognostic models provide patients and their health care providers with general guidelines about how the "average" person fares with the disease, and can be helpful particularly when they are interpreted with the understanding that any individual might vary greatly from a calculated average.

Suggested References

Kassirer, J.P., & Kopelman, R.I. (1991). *Learning clinical reasoning.* Baltimore: Williams & Wilkins. This book covers both diagnostic and therapeutic reasoning. Its strengths lie in the extensive attention given to the role of uncertainty in making clinical decisions, as well as its unique structure: The first part of the book provides detailed discussions of such concepts as cognitive errors and biases in decision making and a cogent argument for problem-based learning. The second part of the book utilizes

60 actual cases, including transcripts of the reasoning processes articulated by expert physicians, to reinforce the concepts introduced earlier in the book.

Petitti, D.B. (1994). *Meta-analysis, decision analysis and cost-effectiveness analysis: Methods for quantitative synthesis in medicine.* Oxford: Oxford Universitiy Press. This text focuses on three of the most important techniques for summarizing data, synthesizing results from numerous studies, and weighing trade-offs associated with different courses of medical action. The approach taken by the author is conceptual rather than highly mathematical. While it is a sophisticated book, it is also extremely readable. The book does a particularly good job outlining the three techniques mentioned in the title, providing examples of each from relevant literature, and assessing the strengths and weaknesses of each method.

Weinstein, M.C., & Fineberg, H.V. (1980). *Clinical decision analysis.* Philadelphia: W.B. Saunders Company. This book is the classic in medical applications of decision analysis. It provides step-by-step instructions on setting up a decision model, selecting probability estimates, and assigning utility values, as well as a balanced discussion of the comparative advantages and shortcomings of the approach. This is a "can't do without" book for anyone contemplating research using decision analysis techniques. However, for readers who are not well-versed in medical terminology and basic concepts of clinical medicine, a medical dictionary and basic text on general internal medicine will prove helpful. This text also provides a good discussion of ROC curves.

Citations In Text

Colditz, G. A., Brewer, T. F., Berkey, C. S., Wilson, M. E., et al. (1994). Efficacy of BCG vaccine in the prevention of tuberculosis. *JAMA, 271,* 698–702.

Early Breast Cancer Trialists' Collaborative Group. (1992). Systemic treatment of early breast cancer by hormonal, cytotoxic, or immune therapy. *Lancet, 339*(8784), 1–15, 71–85.

Jordan, T. J., Grallo, R., & Montgomery, R. (1994). Combining decision analysis and experimental data: The example of benign prostatic hypertrophy. *Journal of Research in Education, 4*(1), 58–67.

Jordan, T. J., Lewit, E., & Reichman, L. B. (1991). Isoniazid preventive therapy for tuberculosis: A decision analysis considering ethnicity and gender. *American Review of Respiratory Disease, 144,* 1357–1360.

Kassirer, J., Alan, J., Moskowitz, J., Lau, J., & Pauker, S. (1987). Decision analysis: A progress report. *Ann Intern Med, 106,* 275–91.

Kopanoff, D. E., Snider, D. E., & Caras, G. J. (1978). Isoniazid-related hepatitis: A U.S. Public Health Service cooperative surveillance study. *American Review of Respiratory Disease, 117,* 991–1001.

National Center for Health Statistics. (1994). *Health, United States, 1993.* Hyattsville, MD: Public Health Service.

Rose, D. N., Schechter, C. B., & Silver, A. L. (1986). The age threshold for isoniazid chemoprophylaxis: A decision analysis for low-risk tuberculin reactors. *JAMA, 256,* 2709–2713.

Sainfort, F. (1991). Evaluation of medical technologies: A generalized ROC analysis. *Medical Decision Making, 11,* 208–220.

Snider, D. E. (1988). Decision analysis for isoniazid preventive therapy: Take it or leave it? *American Review of Respiratory Disease, 137,* 2–3.

Steering Committee of the Physicians' Health Study Research Group. (1989). Final report on the aspirin component of the ongoing physicians' health study. *N Engl J Med, 321*(26), 1825–1828.

Taylor, W. C., Aronson, M. D., & Delbanco, T. L. (1981). Should young adults with a positive tuberculin test take isoniazid? *Ann Intern Med, 94,* 808–813.

Tsevat, J., Taylor, W. C., Wong, J. B., & Pauker, S. G. (1988). Isoniazid for the tuberculin reactor: Take it or leave it. *American Review of Respiratory Disease, 137,* 215–220.

7

Chapter Seven

Medical Information in Cyberspace

Philosophy is written in this grand book, the universe, which stands continually open to our gaze, but the book cannot be understood unless one first learns to comprehend the language and read the letters in which it is composed . . . without these, one wanders about in a dark labyrinth.

Galileo

There is no prescription I can give you more valuable than knowledge.

C. Everett Koop

Introduction

Cyberspace is a term introduced by the novelist William Gibson, and currently is used to refer to the vast range of resources available through computer networks. The network known today as the Internet is a global computer network that emerged during the 1960s as a United States military project to serve as a fall-back for sharing information in the event of a nuclear strike. The Internet combines information management systems and communications systems with the powerful effect of delivering information with unprecedented speed and volume. The introduction of the World Wide Web two decades after the beginnings of the Internet provided a user-friendly, standardized way in which the general public could tap the resources of the global network. The combination of the Internet and the World Wide Web has been a social as well as a technological triumph, since this duo has opened vast warehouses of knowledge to virtually anyone who has access to a computer and a communication line.

The developers of the Web intended it to be "a pool of human knowledge, which would allow collaborators in remote sites to share ideas and all aspects of a common project" (Bereners-Lee et al., 1994). But the Web triggered Internet use far beyond forecasters expectations: "The Web permits users to navigate easily across the global Internet. Here they can view a bewildering variety of information, from the bizarre and inaccurate, to the most up-to-date information available from scientific bodies, newspapers and academic journals" (Coiera, 1997).

The great social value of the Web/Internet combination lies in providing lay people access to information which, not so long ago, was the purview of privileged individuals in academia, government, and selected professions. When the walls of the ivory towers crumbled and equal access to information became possible, problems emerged in evaluating the worth of what was retrieved. The Internet yields information in many different forms, including raw data, peer-reviewed articles, and discussions in "chat rooms." Material obtained from a search of the Internet can run the gamut from completely informal comments to heavily synthesized and formally analyzed information. Knowing how much confidence to have in what one has retrieved, and how to retrieve something in which one can have confidence, are central problems in information consumerism. What is unique to the Internet is the sheer amount of information readily available to the user and, with it, virtually boundless opportunity to be mislead if the information being consumed is not subjected to rigorous scrutiny.

In the health care arena, the Internet has achieved the goal of empowering patients to work in tandem with their physicians in the pursuit of better outcomes. In a popular book aimed at consumers of health care information, Ferguson (1996, p. vii) provided the following example:

"When Sara Style's doctor prescribed Cotrimoxazole for her recurring bladder infections, Sara went right home, logged on to Prodigy, and read a detailed profile of the drug in the Consumer Reports Drug Database. To her surprise, she discovered that Cotrimoxazole (a combination of the antibiotic drugs sulfamethoxazole and trimethoprim) could interact with the blood thinner, Coumadin, which she was taking to prevent blood clots in her legs. This combination could have produced a potentially fatal hemorrhage. She also learned that the drug could produce skin rashes, itching, or severe sunburn after only a few minutes' exposure to sunlight—and Sara was an avid gardener. She immediately e-mailed her doctor, enclosing copies of her findings, and suggested that a single dose of amoxicillin (which, according to her online research, posed fewer problems) might be a better choice. Sara's doctor agreed, phoned in the new prescription to Sara's local pharmacy, and sent Sara an e-mail thanking her for helping to avoid the potential problems."

At first pass, this case reads like an advertisement for the positive powers of information, with patient and physician working interactively to decide upon an optimal treatment regimen. Read more critically, however, it becomes a story without an ending. Amoxicillin is a notoriously poor treatment choice for bladder infections, ergo the selection of a combination of sulfamethoxazole and trimethoprim. What happened to Sara's bladder infection? What was the likelihood of successful treatment with amoxicillin? And what were the odds of a serious drug interaction with Coumadin? If Sara's organism proved unresponsive to amoxicillin, was she confronted with the necessity of taking Cotrimoxazole anyway? And, on a more general level, how "good" is the information provided in the Consumer Reports Drug Database? Who provides information to this database—the drug companies who market treatment products or third-party evaluators?

Much of what is written about the Internet is technologically oriented, with how-to's aimed at getting the user familiar with tools for accessing material. Such resources are necessary, but they are outdated almost as soon as they are written, and they target techniques in the absence of a critical framework for structuring an Internet search and evaluating what the search generates. The goal of this chapter is to provide a framework that can be used to formulate Internet search strategies and to assess the value, from personal as well as scientific perspectives, of medical information obtained in cyberspace. First, the levels at which information exists are discussed with attention to the amount of processing and interpreting what has occurred before the material reaches the consumer. Distinctions are made among data, information, and knowledge. Second, examples are used to illustrate concretely the process of deconstructing knowledge obtained from the Internet. Attention is focused on the judgments that are made at each step in the process. The chapter concludes with suggested guidelines for using the Internet well and for identifying the strengths and weaknesses of Internet-based information.

Levels of Information in Cyberspace

Information tends to drive out knowledge. Information is just signs and numbers, while knowledge has semantic value. What we want is knowledge, but what we often get is information. It is a sign of the times that many people cannot tell the difference between information and knowledge, not to mention wisdom, which even knowledge tends sometimes to drive out.

Heinz Pagels

■DATA, INFORMATION, AND KNOWLEDGE

Throughout this book, the word *information* has been used in a general way to refer to the content of communications about health care, including risks and benefits of diagnostic and treatment modalities, likelihood of diseases, and estimates of the health of population groups. Medical information is communicated in language that relies heavily on numbers, particularly in the form of probabilities.

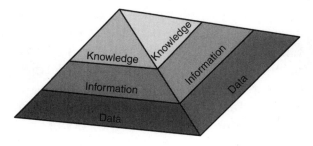

Figure 7a Hierarchy of meaning.

In the specialty known as information science, and in the design of information systems such as the Internet, the word *information* is defined more precisely. Distinctions are made among three related terms: data, information, and knowledge. These three terms comprise what is conceptualized as a hierarchy of meaning (Coiera, 1997), which can be represented as a pyramid (Figure 7a).

This more precise conceptualization becomes helpful when a consumer attempts to assess the degree of confidence that can be had in material retrieved from cyberspace.

Data are at the foundation of meaning and the core of the scientific method. Typically, data are thought of as "facts" such as a patient's biological gender, blood pressure, T-cell count, HIV viral load, etc. Data can exist in **raw** form, meaning that nothing has been done in terms of alteration or modification. In order to form databases that can be analyzed statistically, raw data sometime require coding. For example, for most statistical programs to "understand" patient's gender, a numerical coding scheme must be used. Female could be coded arbitrarily as 1 and male as 0. Regardless of the fact that coding has been done, gender remains at the level of data.

Information exists when data are placed in a context that provides meaning. Clancy (1995, p. 229) states that "information is constructed by people in a process of perception." If a patient's blood pressure is measured at 180/95 mmHg, this piece of data is likely to inform the clinician that the patient requires management of hypertension. In this example, the clinician's perception of the data raises the "fact" of a blood pressure measurement to the next level in the hierarchy–information. In order for blood pressure data to become information, the clinician has interpreted a fact in the context of medical literature about hypertension. So, one way to grasp the concept of information is to think of it as data that have been put into a context. This contextualization may occur through the perceptions of experts or the application of statistical programs. What is important to remember about information is that it has already been contextualized: Someone or something has processed/interpreted data in order to create meaning. The information consumer must be aware of the adequacy of the processing/interpreting that has been done in order to decide whether to accept the meaning that has been assigned to the data.

An example of contextualizing data from two opposite vantage points is provided in the following Statistical Assessment Service report, obtained as an online service. The lead question, "What's a parent to think?" encapsulates the problem of contextualized data in a news report on infant deaths. Consumers of information would do well to consider: Who's context is it, anyway?

Right Report, Wrong Headline

What's a parent to think? A Sept. 25th USA Today article headlined "Decline in infant deaths masks troubling factors" actually contains a lot of good news. The infant mortality rate has fallen again, as has the rate of infant deaths from birth defects. Yet the downbeat headline dwells on the higher proportion of all deaths caused by birth defects.

Fatalities owing to birth defects actually fell from 255 per 100,000 in 1980 to 168 per 100,000 in 1995. Because this rate has fallen more slowly than the overall infant mortality rate, however, the proportion of infant deaths attributable to birth defects has risen.

Journalists seem able to find something depressing in the happiest of stories. But this is all good news. A better headline would have been "Medical advances help more infants live."

Knowledge is the part of the pyramid where most meaning-making occurs. There are many different philosophical approaches to attaining knowledge. From the perspective of contemporary medicine, knowledge typically is thought of as the attainment of general rules that, hopefully, are "true."

Knowledge provides ways in which information can be processed and contexualized. Coiera (1997, pp. 17–19) states that: "Knowledge can now be recognized to be the set of models we have built up to understand and interact with the world. . . . Healthcare is an information and knowledge intensive activity. Data are constantly being gathered, and their meaning evaluated against a set of models. . . a model that contains knowledge about the way concepts are related is needed to draw inferences based upon the data.

At the level of knowledge, material has been contextualized in a formal way, relations among phenomena have been described, and meaning has been assigned based on an existing model. Before the discovery of microbes, surgeons took no precautions for sterilization. Anecdotes have been told about surgeons appearing at the operating table in street clothes, with unwashed hands, flicking cigar ashes on the floor of the operating theater. Post-surgical mortality was "understood" as an unavoidable correlate of the body undergoing surgery—because the existing "knowledge" was a model in which people died from the trauma of surgery and did not include a model of avoidable infection. When microbes were discovered, and the presence of microbes was linked to infection from surgical procedures, some basic knowledge about the workings of infectious organisms and the need for sterilization was attained. This knowledge contributed greatly to a reduction in mortality. This example illustrates that not all of what is thought of as knowledge is, in fact, true. When knowledge is mistaken for truth, data and information can be processed in dangerously misleading ways.

■INTERRELATIONS AMONG DATA, INFORMATION, AND KNOWLEDGE

As more is learned about medicine and health care, models are enhanced, rejected, and sometimes replaced by new models that reflect better our understanding of the natural world. Data, information, and knowledge are interrelated in ways that are complex and sometimes difficult to identify. For example, knowledge can affect data because scientists typically look for phenomena they expect to find and do not look for things that are beyond the scope of the models that inform their work. Also, data "drive" the development of models, so that relations among phenomena that serve as the foundation of knowledge are only as good as the data from which they are developed. Sometimes, great advances in science occur when accidental findings that do not fit existing models are studied in depth instead of thrown out as error. Fleming's work leading to the discovery of penicillin is an example of an accidental discovery.

Before the idea of microbes arose, and before the microscope was developed, scientists did not look for microorganisms in patients who had severe fever and other symptoms of illness after surgery. Once a model of infectious microorganisms was developed, scientists began attempts to identify and catalogue types of organisms, as well as to find ways to avoid and to treat infections. Going in the other direction, data affect knowledge because data reveal relationships upon which models are built. In the early years of investigation of HIV disease, most data were derived from populations in which sexual contact was the primary route of disease transmission. Models of the disease were developed that presented it as a sexually transmitted disease. Later, HIV disease was identified in patients who used intravenous drugs and, apparently, contracted the virus from contaminated blood products during needle sharing. Data from these populations expanded the model of HIV beyond that of a sexually transmitted disease.

Because it is contextualized, information is never completely "objective"—it has been processed in some way, often through the application of knowledge. During the early 1980s, a patient who appeared in an urban emergency room with data including high fever of unknown origin, history of dramatic and unwanted weight loss, and swollen lymph glands, often was diagnosed as having some kind of influenza. Later in that decade, the same data were likely to be contextualized using the knowledge that had been attained regarding HIV (then referred to only as AIDS). In this new context, the data were likely to be understood as information about the possibility that the patient was infected with HIV. Information can be thought of as the contextualization of data through the use of existing knowledge. A fundamental purpose for consulting a physician when one is experiencing symptoms is the anticipation that the physician will apply his/her knowledge to the data (symptoms) to make meaning of what is happening.

■SEARCHING LEVELS OF THE CYBERSPACE PYRAMID

A user seeking an answer to a medical question on the Internet may start at any of the three levels of the pyramid described above. What is retrieved might range from rigorously reviewed scientific sources to personal, anecdotal opinions. The question the user is asking dictates the kinds of sources searched. The way the answers will be used dictates the amount of rigor that will be required in the material that is retrieved. Following are two linked examples of questions and possible methods for obtaining answers using the Internet.

Example 1

A medical oncologist has been following a 55-year-old woman with a family history of breast cancer for the past 10 years. The patient's most recent mammogram showed a pattern of diffuse, calcified lesions. On biopsy, these lesions were identified as *lobular carcinoma in situ (LCIS)*. The physician is aware that some controversy has existed regarding the treatment of a patient with this finding. This type of lesion is encapsulated and does not show the pattern of spread that characterizes "true" breast cancer. In other words, it has been regarded as a benign lesion. On the other hand, this lesion seems to have acted as a "marker" for a higher risk of developing the types of breast lesions that metastasize and become life threatening. The physician's question is: *To maximize this patient's life expectancy given her biopsy findings, should the medical recommendation be regular follow-up mammograms at frequent intervals or should she undergo preventive mastectomy?*

Search Strategy: The Internet search begins at the top—at the level of knowledge. The physician queries most recent textbooks and journal articles in peer-reviewed publications. She finds that while preventive mastectomy had been the treatment of choice for many decades since the 1940s, the advent of mammography heralded an era in which intensive screening was used in lieu of surgery for this finding. The present recommendation appears to be to follow with screening rather than perform surgery. However, the physician detects equivocal arguments in these knowledge sources. For example, while screening is preferred to surgery, sources indicate that a very high risk patient history could alter the recommendation.

The physician also checks material she has obtained from *Medscape,* which provides frequent updates via e-mail of current research issues as well as links to the sources of the information. *Medscape* resides at the top of the pyramid because it contains information that has been highly processed using knowledge from various medical specialties. However, the links it provides can take the physician to other levels of the pyramid.

After her search at the level of knowledge, the physician remains uncertain about the optimal course of action for her patient. She embarks on a process of moving down into the pyramid, a process called following a thread. To follow a thread, the user moves from the knowledge level of cyberspace into information and perhaps into data levels (which might or might not be available). By getting closer to the data, she will be in an increasingly better position to evaluate whether to accept the conclusions presented in the form of knowledge at higher levels in cyberspace. Following a thread can be a difficult process because as the user moves from a point atop the pyramid to somewhere deeper within its structure, there will be many possible paths to follow. One of the most common problems encountered in following a thread is getting lost while surfing the Web.

In this instance, the physician wishes to view actual data obtained from women who had been diagnosed with lobular carcinoma *in situ*. As she queries the Internet for databases, she locates *SEER,* a program of the National Cancer Institute that collects and publishes cancer incidence and survival data from cancer registries from the U.S. population. Accessing *SEER,* the physician can begin to view data that bear closely on the case she is treating. She finds, in particular, a longitudinal database from the state of Connecticut that was developed to follow women diagnosed with lobular carcinoma *in situ* over the course of their lives.

At the level of the data available from the Connecticut registry, the thread stops. The physician can find no additional links of good quality. She decides to look closely at the data available from this registry to determine whether it can assist her in her treatment recommendation.

In this example, the physician will need many skills to use the Internet to assist her to arrive at an optimal recommendation. First, she will need to be clear about the process of following a thread, beginning at the level of knowledge and digging as deeply as necessary without getting lost or side-tracked on the Internet. Getting lost could mean failing to find links to the *SEER* database, for example. Second, she will need to be skilled in evaluating not only the quality of the studies presented at the levels of both knowledge and information, but will need also the skills to evaluate the quality of a database once she has arrived at the deepest levels of the pyramid. Because this user will integrate the material she retrieves from her Internet search into a health care recommendation for a patient with a potentially serious condition, she will focus her efforts on the best research investigations she can find as well as the most complete and accurate data.

What she has not utilized in this search process are informal systems such as chat rooms, since she has been seeking material that is scientifically based rather than personal or anecdotal.

Example 2

The 55-year old woman who has received a diagnosis of lobular carcinoma *in situ* from her physician (in Example 1 above) is experiencing confusion and concern. She has read literature provided to her by her physician. The explanations of her diagnosis and possible treatment options seem to leave room for her to exercise her preferences. However, the medical literature has not provided resources to help her project what it would be like living with this diagnosis and the associated frequent checks for cancer. Although her mother and sister have undergone surgery and chemotherapy for breast cancer, they were diagnosed with metastatic disease. If she were to elect preventive mastectomy, she would not require chemotherapy or the lymph node dissections that were necessary for her mother and sister. This woman's questions are: What is it like, on a personal level, to live with the diagnosis of lobular carcinoma in situ? What is it like to have this threat hanging over you or, on the other hand, to remove the threat by electing preventive mastectomy?

Search Strategy: The questions this woman is posing will not be answered by large-scale investigations that crunch numbers to arrive at something like average quality-of-life ratings. Instead, she is looking for qualitative reflections from the personal perspectives of individual women. She knows that lobular carcinoma *in situ* is relatively rare, so her chances of finding women with this diagnosis through avenues other than the Internet are slim. Her hope is that by locating women on the Internet who are willing to share their experiences with her, she will be able better to sort out what she is facing as well as to clarify her personal preferences for treatment.

In terms of a search strategy, this woman is most likely to find the material she seeks at the level of information. She is not searching for data, but rather for data put into context to provide meaning. Said differently, she is looking for the meaning individual women have made of their diagnosis and treatments, the ways they have contextualized the fact of lobular carcinoma *in situ* in their lives. Some options open to her are chat rooms, on-line support groups, cancer-related organizations with patient information and communication links, and open searches using key words that will "hit" areas of the Internet frequented by women with her diagnosis.

It may seem that this user's job lies mainly in retrieving information with little attention to evaluating the quality of the information she receives. The situation can be quite the reverse of this expectation. Unlike the material contained in scientific sites or national health databases, the personal information sought by this user does not need to meet any requirements to be posted on the Internet. Unlike the scientific sites, there is no oversight body to evaluate the credentials of experts making claims about diagnoses and treatments, or guidelines by which to evaluate the quality of a research study or the representativeness of a database. In her search to find out how others have made meaning of the experience of lobular carcinoma *in situ,* she may retrieve information that helps her better to cope with her diagnosis as well as information that confuses and concerns her even more.

For the kind of qualitative material sought by the patient in this example, it is nearly impossible to set criteria for good versus bad information. Perhaps the patient will find comfort in an e-mail response from a woman who has had this diagnosis for 10 years, has not developed breast cancer, and who believes that follow-up screenings are unnecessary. Her quality of life has been fine, she has been untroubled by thoughts of cancer, and has not incurred the inconvenience or the expense of screening. The advice imbedded in this information is in contradiction to the best medical advice available which, at a basic minimum, suggests routine screening. In addition to the above perspective, the patient seeking information might retrieve the story of a woman who complied with a rigorous screening regimen, developed invasive cancer that was diagnosed too late to achieve a cure, and is suffering the terminal stages of disease. Her quality of life is miserable, she has undergone surgeries that were not curative, and she is experiencing the worst aspects of heroic courses of chemotherapy. Seen from this context, aggressive surgery to prevent invasive disease could appear to be the only sensible approach.

One of the great difficulties inherent in retrieving personal, qualitative information from the Internet to inform medical decisions is that even questions aimed at understanding what it is like to live with a diagnosis invariably contain covert if not overt medical "advice." One guideline that might help in soliciting qualitative information via the Internet is to sample widely and thereby avoid getting caught up in a single source (such as one chat room, or the communications link of one organization) which might be more likely to present a view from only one context. To understand better the personal experience of living with lobular carcinoma *in situ*, having the experience contextualized from diverse vantage points is likely to provide something closest to reality.

Deconstructing Knowledge from the Internet and the Example of Health Care Ratings

■DECONSTRUCTION

Deconstructing means taking something apart, separating it into its elemental pieces, and evaluating the validity of these pieces. The ideas of deconstructionism originated in attempts to take apart the texts produced by researchers (primarily in the social sciences) in order to scrutinize the material for the researcher's biases, unstated assumptions, and interpretations of events, in the anticipation that alternate ways of looking at the data might be possible (Derrida, 1976; Clough, 1998).

Applying a form of deconstructionism to knowledge obtained from the Internet is appealing because the sheer volume of available material coupled with the absence of censorship applied to much of the material paves the way for biases, founded and unfounded assumptions, and varied interpretations. The purpose of deconstructing Internet-based knowledge is to assess the status of retrievable knowledge in a particular topic area. One begins with what might appear to be objective truth and follows a process of deconstruction to understand how this knowledge has come to be regarded as true or at least reasonable. In this process, something that has been presented as an objective truth might come to be seen as true only under certain conditions, true for some people but not for others, or perhaps, not true at all. The deconstruction process discussed in this section is most appropriate to material obtained from formal information systems, in which the user seeks scientifically based knowledge.

What is somewhat paradoxical about material obtained from the Internet is that it bombards us in large volumes from many sources. Different forms of Internet "media" are vying for our attention almost constantly and often simultaneously. Yet, the knowledge we adopt as seemingly most relevant or truthful often is presented in a highly compressed form. The knowledge **bite** that sets the course for deconstruction is very likely to come from an Internet source—but it might impinge in another form of media, as in the example that follows in this chapter.

Regardless of how the initial bite trapped our attention, we typically use the Internet to follow through on finding out more about it. If the bite comes from the Internet, it is likely to have originated somewhere close to the top of the information pyramid. Regardless of the initial source, a knowledge bite is a highly processed and highly synthesized abstract or summary of material contained in a much larger body of knowledge.

When the user intends to base an important decision on the knowledge bite, or wishes to be certain that what is being learned is correct for any number of reasons, the validity of what is being claimed should be evaluated. Because evaluating knowledge on the Internet differs in some respects from evaluating knowledge from more traditional sources, going through a process of deconstruction can be helpful.

While deconstruction as it is practiced in other fields focuses on "taking apart" material, deconstruction applied to knowledge available on the Internet often requires an expansion of the material that will be used in the deconstruction process. Keeping this in mind, what is suggested here is a deconstruction process comprised of the following three steps:

1. Expanding the knowledge bite by locating original source materials and related references.
2. Validating the knowledge bite by verifying that the source documents support the facts and conclusions presented, that the sources contain no critical errors, and that the sources have not been superceded (i.e., outdated) by other developments in the field.
3. Developing a critical understanding of the context in which the knowledge exists and recontextualizing it if necessary to help ensure that the conclusions, recommendations, or policy decisions are not exaggerations or projections unsupported by the data in the original sources.

The following example illustrates the application of these steps.

■FOLLOWING THE PROCESS OF DECONSTRUCTION THROUGH THE EXAMPLE OF HEALTH CARE RATINGS

The knowledge bite: A brief response recorded in an interview on public health

An interview with Dr. C. Everett Koop was published in the January–February 2001 issue of the *Dartmouth Alumni Maga-*

zine. The interview was conducted and reported by Dr. Julie Low, a physician and a resident in training in psychiatry. The interview introduced Dr. Koop as an alumnus of Dartmouth College, class of 1937, a graduate of Cornell Medical School, former chief of surgery at Children's Hospital of Philadelphia, a pioneer in pediatric surgery, and U.S. Surgeon General from 1981 to 1988. These credentials lend credibility to his knowledge of health care. The knowledge bite of interest in this example is Dr. Koop's response to a report issued recently by the World Health Organization (WHO) about the quality of health care worldwide:

> Q. (Dr. Low) Did you see the WHO study that rated the health-care systems of different countries in terms of satisfaction? The United States was way down on the list.
>
> A. (Dr. Koop) We were No. 37, but you have to be careful about such surveys. One of the things they use in all those rating studies is infant mortality. If a baby is a stillborn in this country, he gets a birth certificate and a death certificate. So there is a birth and there is a death and that is a mortality. But in many countries, stillborns are not counted, so their infant mortality rate appears much lower than ours. So you have to question how they get their statistics. Another question to ask is, not which country has the best care, but which country would you most like to get sick in? I think a lot of people would say, no matter what my country rating is, I would like to be sick in the United States.

The knowledge bite provided by Dr. Koop contains two parts. The first part targets the use of different approaches to reporting infant mortality in different countries that biases the rating against the United States. The second part states Dr. Koop's opinion that people in the United States prefer the care they receive here over care available elsewhere. Dr. Koop has responded to a part of a statement released by the WHO. He has elected to respond by focusing only on infant mortality, and he contextualizes his comments with the statement that people would rather get sick "here" regardless of the rating. To deconstruct Dr. Koop's responses, the user must expand the knowledge base to include material from the WHO report itself. Second, the systematic bias he identifies in infant mortality ratings needs validating, as does his statement about the central role of infant mortality in the overall rating of health care. Third, the context in which he views the WHO statements should be evaluated to assess the extent to which this context might distort his processing of the information.

Step 1: Expanding the Knowledge

To expand this knowledge bite to a knowledge base, Internet searching yielded the following relevant materials:

- The World Health Organization Web site provides the full version of the official Press Release.
- The World Health Organization Web site provides a full text version of the report from which the Press Release was generated: *The World Health Report 2000—Health Systems: Improving Performance.*
- The World Health Organization Web site provides access to sets of statistical tables that were used to compile the Report.
- The World Health Organization Web site also provides online assistance for access to a traditional database that was not used specifically in compiling the Report referred to above, but which provides additional information about data collection/measurement protocols.

Step 2: Validating the Knowledge

The Press Release: Excerpts from the Full Text In the following excerpts, particularly relevant sections are underlined.

World Health Organization Assesses the World's Health Systems

The World Health Organization has carried out the first ever analysis of the world's health systems. <u>Using five performance indicators</u> to measure health systems in 191 member states, it finds that France provides the best overall health care followed among major countries by Italy, Spain, Oman,

Austria and Japan. The findings are published today, 21 June, in The World Health Report 2000—Health systems: Improving performance.

The U.S. health system spends a higher portion of its gross domestic product than any other country but ranks 37 out of 191 countries according to its performance, the report finds. The United Kingdom, which spends just six percent of GDP on health services, ranks 18th. Several small countries—San Marino, Andorra, Malta and Singapore are rated close behind second-placed Italy.

In designing the framework for health system performance, WHO broke new methodological ground, employing a technique not previously used for health systems. It compares each country's system to what the experts estimate to be the upper limit of what can be done with the level of resources available in that country. It also measures what each country's system has accomplished in comparison with those of other countries.

WHO's assessment system was based on five indicators: overall level of population health; health inequalities (or disparities) within the population; overall level of health system responsiveness (a combination of patient satisfaction and how well the system acts); distribution of responsiveness within the population (how well people of varying economic status find that they are served by the health system); and the distribution of the health system's financial burden within the population (who pays the costs).

Dr. Koop appears to have responded to the correct press release, since he stated that it rated the United States in 37th place. Dr. Koop did not state that their were five indicators that were used for the rating. In these indicators, there is no mention of infant mortality at all. If it is used to comprise one of the indices, and if it is in fact biased against the United States, this is not apparent from the official Press Release. Thus, there is no indication in the Press Release that data collection mechanisms that overreport infant mortality in the United States existed, or that such over reporting would effect a change from 37th place. (A user who is somewhat versed in contemporary health policy might consider that other factors, such as patient satisfaction, appear in more than one indicator, as do distribution of services, inequality or disparity of service, and economic status. These issues are of concern to the U.S. public and are publicly debated everyday. The high cost of prescription drugs and health care for the underserved urban and rural poor, the elderly, and children in poverty are ongoing and unresolved issues that are likely to impact heavily on the indices.)

Excerpts from the Full Report and Protocol Descriptions of WHO Data In addition to the Press Release, the search yielded information about the nature of the data used in the Release. The first excerpts that follow are from a special database that was generated from 191 countries using several new indices to develop perspectives on world health. This formed the basis of the Press Release and report referred to earlier.

> Health is the defining objective for the health system. This means making the health status of the entire population as good as possible over people's whole life cycle, taking account of both premature mortality and disability. Annex Table 2 presents three conventional and partial measures of health status, by country, without ranking: these are the probability of dying before age 5 years or between ages 15 and 59 years, and life expectancy at birth. For the first time these measures are presented with estimates of uncertainty, and these uncertainties carry over to subsequent calculations. On the basis of the mortality figures, five strata are identified, ranging from low child and adult mortality to high child mortality and very high adult death rates. Combining these strata with the six WHO Regions gives 14 subregions defined geographically and epidemiologically (see the list of Member States by WHO Region and mortality stratum). Annex Table 3 presents estimates of mortality by cause and sex in 1999 in each of these subregions (not by country), and Annex Table 4 combines these death rates with information about disability to create estimates of one measure of overall population health: the burden of disease, that is, the numbers of disability-adjusted life years (DALYs) lost.

From the above excerpts, we see that the Report utilized new methods for calculating life expectancy, with attention to child mortality. The user could also go to the Annex Tables to view the specific statistics referred to in the Report.

In contrast, the following excerpt retrieved from the Internet is from the traditional WHO database that is comprised of input from 80 countries. It appears most likely that Dr. Koop had this database in mind when he made his response.

The World Health Organization's Mortality Database

. . . The age groups employed vary by country and may vary for one country over time. Countries may group deaths according to 5-year (or 10-year) age groups between 5 and 9 (or 5 and 14) years and from 60 to 64 (or 55 to 64) years. Age groups under 5 years of age are variable; some countries use age 0 and age 1–4 years grouped, and others use age 0 and years 1, 2, 3, 4 in single years. Similarly, the existence and grouping of death data for the population over 64 varies: deaths to the older population exist grouped for all ages 65 and over, 70 and over, 75 and over, or 85 and over. Furthermore, there are combinations of the different groupings for the youngest and oldest ages: at present 9 age codes exist in the data base, including deaths provided without reference to age. <u>Finally, the ages employed to classify infant deaths—deaths at age 0 years—also vary, in particular for the neonatal period: deaths may or may not be separately reported that occurred in the first 28 days, whereas in some cases, neonatal reports are complete for deaths on day 0, in week 1 (days 1 to 6), in the first four weeks (days 7–27), or subsequently (days 28–364).</u>

Dr. Koop correctly stated that there are differences in the protocol for reporting infant mortality in the survey data collected.

Step 3: Understanding the Context and Recontextualizing the Knowledge If Necessary

At this point in the process, several conclusions can be drawn:

1. At the time of the interview, Dr. Koop knew that WHO had issued a Press Release and/or a Report. This is based on his correctly placing the United States as 37th.
2. The answer was accurate insofar as it described an inherent bias in one aspect of the traditional WHO data-

base, which was superseded by the new Report that used special measures. While Dr. Koop's emphasis on infant mortality raises a legitimate bias issue, it is not clearly related to the new Report.

3. Dr. Koop did not mention any of the other indicators used in the new WHO Report or the impact other factors such as patient satisfaction apparently exerted on the rating.
4. Dr. Koop's answer seemed to suggest that if only infant mortality were measured according to a standardized system, the U.S. rating would be much higher.

In terms of context, Dr. Koop linked his statement about U.S. ratings to infant mortality data. Looking back at the introductory description of his background, we see an emphasis on pediatric care and pediatric surgery, which accounts for this context. In addition, Dr. Koop appeared to have perceived the material from the context of the traditional WHO database rather than the new Report. Consequently, Dr. Koop contextualized the WHO statements about U.S. health care using his frame of pediatrics—a more narrow frame than the target of the status of U.S. health care in general and framed his views on the basis of the traditional rather than the new WHO reporting system. He included a statement of opinion that people would rather get sick in the U.S. regardless of the rating provided by the WHO. This contextualization clearly lets the user know that Dr. Koop favors U.S. health care. His point of reference for this opinion includes vast experience and clearly places again another of his own contexts on the WHO findings. What he essentially is doing is taking U.S. health care out of the context of the WHO report, and recontextualizing it using his own experiential frame of reference. The problem confronting the user of this "knowledge" is whether to accept the contexts Dr. Koop has used or to recontextualize it using a different frame, such as the satisfaction and access oriented frame adopted by WHO. Here is another way the information bite that began this process could look if the WHO context had been used:

Alternate perspective: We were 37th, and this was based on five indicators that focused heavily on patient satisfaction and their perceptions of ease of access to service. These are issues that are in the forefront of public debates regarding U.S. health care, so it is not surprising that these would surface in the type of data collected by the WHO. From examination of the measurement and data collection in the special WHO report, one could conclude that the rating is possibly an accurate measure of what the WHO set out to investigate. On the other hand, if other measures of health care had been utilized, the rating received by the U.S. might have been different.

■SUMMARY OF THE DECONSTRUCTION PROCESS

At the end of this process, the user might or might not elect to accept the knowledge bite in its original form. What has occurred, however, is a developed awareness of the points at which this knowledge bite represents or fails to represent the larger knowledge base from which it was drawn, as well as a sensitivity to the contextualization that framed the knowledge bite. The consumer of this material is now in a far better position to decide which form of knowledge bite makes most sense to incorporate in decision making or in augmenting one's own knowledge.

Adventures in Cyberspace: Some Guidelines for Using the Internet as a Medical Resource

We live in a time when we have access, literally, to the entire Library of Congress on our desktops. In the roles of both health care providers and health care consumers, we can obtain volumes of health information and support online at any time of the day or night, at little or no cost. In addition to formal communications such as online journal articles, research reports, and textbooks, we can communicate with others who are willing to share experiences and lend support to our struggles.

However, the reality is that given good Internet search tools and the know-how to use them, we are likely to be able to access far more material than we possibly can consume on most health related topics. If we are acting in the role of a health care provider, we are confronted often with little turn-around time to search for information to assist in making diagnostic or therapeutic recommendations. If we are acting in the role of patient, typically we have limited time within which to make up our minds about a course of medical action. This means that we need to find ways to use the Internet efficiently to retrieve the kinds of materials that are best suited to our needs.

Getting what we need from the Internet on a "real-time" basis requires that we do three things:

1. Decide what use we intend to make of the material we retrieve.
2. Structure a search strategy that will retrieve the kinds of materials that will best meet the needs we have identified.
3. Understand the relative merits of formal versus informal information systems and evaluate each according to appropriate standards.

Most people begin most Internet searches very broadly, for example, by entering some key words such as a diagnosis. Depending to some extent on the software in use and the specific online services subscribed to, broad searches tend to yield many hits spanning many types of material. For the example of lobular carcinoma *in situ* used earlier in this chapter, a broad search using only the diagnostic finding as key words yielded more than 100 hits. These included scholarly sources, cancer news bulletins, support groups, art produced by people with cancer, virtual classrooms, and e-mail conversations with expert oncologists. Following the links provided by each of these hits would increase exponentially the amount of material retrieved. Much of this material would be irrelevant to the purpose of the search, time consuming to sift through, and possibly distracting. The moral of the example is that searching without a clear purpose and strategy can easily get the user lost in cyberspace. The remainder of this section discusses in greater detail the three tasks delineated above.

■ DECIDE WHAT USE WE INTEND TO MAKE OF THE MATERIAL WE RETRIEVE

What is the task we are attempting to accomplish by using the Internet to access medical material?

Some tasks a patient might set for him/herself could include:

- Find out more facts about his/her diagnosis to fill in the gaps in knowledge that remained after discussion with the physician.
- Learn about available treatment options.
- Locate other physicians for the purpose of getting another opinion about treatment.
- Identify an online support group that will provide hints and help for living with a specific medical condition.
- Find out what patients who have gone through a specific therapy think and feel about their experiences.
- Learn what to expect at various points in the clinical course of the disease.
- Find other patients who are willing to correspond outside the structure of a support group.

Some tasks a health care provider might set for him/herself could include:

- Learn about state-of-the-art therapies for treating a particular disease and where the therapies are available.
- Learn from patients in an anonymous "setting" what their experiences of a particular treatment or diagnostic modality have been.
- Identify and confer with other medical experts on a topic that appears equivocal in the medical literature.

- Compare risks of disease at his/her own facility with risks at other sites.
- Find databases relevant to a particular topic that are available for analysis/research purposes.
- Conduct survey research about patient health care preferences using the Internet to obtain the survey sample and administer the questionnaire.
- Find sources for continuing education in subspecialty areas.
- Identify a support group for health care providers who are experiencing burn-out.

When the use we intend to make of the material we retrieve is clear, as in the sample tasks above, the use will provide direction for developing a search strategy. A fundamental clue that the intended use of the material is not yet sufficiently clear is having in mind only a topic, such as a key word, without any questions or goals articulated about the topic.

■ STRUCTURE A SEARCH STRATEGY THAT WILL RETRIEVE THE KINDS OF MATERIALS THAT WILL BEST MEET THE NEEDS WE HAVE IDENTIFIED

Matching how the material is going to be used to the types of sites that are likely to provide the most appropriate and relevant, high-quality material is what frames an Internet search strategy. While this might seem obvious, many if not most Internet users search without a strategy. The result is volumes of largely irrelevant information, inability to follow a thread, absence of planned ways of evaluating retrieved materials, and missed opportunities to move efficiently to the in-depth or specific material that could be most useful.

In the event that the user has no idea what kinds of resources exist on the Internet to meet a particular need, a broad search using key words can be performed for the purpose of mapping the domain of resources. This means getting an overview of what is available while being careful not to lose track of the purpose for conducting the search.

For most topics searched in health care, there are some predictable types of sites that are encountered. These types include the following categories:

- Meta-sources, such as *MedScape,* which provide highly processed and synthesized information.
- Libraries, such as the National Library of Medicine, and the National Library of Congress.
- International health care information groups, such as the World Health Organization.
- National health care groups, such as the National Centers for Disease Control and Prevention, National Cancer Institute, and National Institutes of Health.
- Private organizations with interest in the health care area, including foundations and corporations.
- Database projects such as *SEER* and related statistical resources.
- University/medical school based information services, such as *OncoLink* provided by the University of Pennsylvania Cancer Center.
- Clinical trial information bases enrolling ongoing and newly completed studies.
- News services and news forums.
- Chat rooms.
- Educational services, including virtual classrooms.
- Psychosocial support services.
- Physician and hospital locators.
- Information services provided by particular physicians.
- Medical sites offering diagnosis and treatment services.
- Web sites hosted by private individuals with a special interest.

After deciding which types of sites are most likely to serve the purposes of the search, the second step in developing a search strategy is to set a hierarchy of importance on the types of materials that appear to be available. For example, a physician beginning subspecialty training in infectious diseases might want to learn about the types and efficacies of antiretroviral therapies available for HIV disease. She intends to use the material she retrieves to amplify her growing knowledge base in clinical medicine which, hopefully, will translate into better patient care. She places at the top of her hierarchy sites that will provide knowledge from experts working in the area as well as information from timely, well-designed research investigations. She might place at a lower priority, yet still relevant to her purpose of learning from timely sources, sites that include preliminary results from studies still in progress. Sites that provide raw data not yet analyzed and interpreted by experts are likely to be either excluded from her search or set at a low level in the hierarchy of importance. In contrast, a physician seeking opportunities to perform research using the resources available on the Internet might place sites including raw data at the top level of importance.

■ UNDERSTAND THE RELATIVE MERITS OF FORMAL VERSUS INFORMAL INFORMATION SYSTEMS AND EVALUATE EACH ACCORDING TO APPROPRIATE STANDARDS

Formal information systems in cyberspace are systems in which data are processed or contextualized according to an agreed upon model (Coiera, 1997). An example of a formal information system is the way in which research investigations are held to standards of scientific rigor, typically through the mechanism of peer review. In contrast, informal information systems are not held to a specific model for interpretation and are not "answerable" to externally imposed structures or standards in the ways that characterize formal systems. An example of an informal information system supported on the Internet is the exchange of ideas in an online support group devoted to discussing living with diabetes.

To evaluate material obtained from formal information systems, the user can apply a range of informatics and research design skills, in the same way one would evaluate formal information obtained by physically visiting an academic library and finding a paper copy of a journal article. There is a long history of accepted ways of doing scientific research and of adhering to appropriate scientific, professional, and ethical standards in the conduct of that research. What is different about tapping formal information systems using the Internet is the sheer volume of material one can obtain with extraordinary speed and convenience.

The Internet provides an infrastructure that supports the exchange of informal information in an unprecedented manner. Prior to the availability of this infrastructure, informal information systems existed only insofar as individuals could locate other individuals willing to share ideas in person, by telephone, or through paper correspondence. There is no history of quality control for the kind of information exchange implemented through the Internet. Additionally, most Internet users would argue strongly for keeping some avenues of communication exempt from formal strictures and retaining the freedom to communicate with the vast audiences connected through the new technologies.

In his enthusiastic support for the infrastructure that makes exchange of informal information possible on such a vast scale, Ferguson (1996, p. 43) talked about *cyberspace friends* and *online angels*. He highlighted the advantages of being able to access support around the clock from individuals who are willing to provide information, sympathy, practical advice, and encouragement. A striking example of what can be accomplished using the Internet is his mention of an online memorial service. While Ferguson had high praise for the self-help capabilities in cyberspace, he paused to note that there are two things these informal systems will not do: "Take on the mantle of the health professional and tell you what to do. [and] Charge you a fee for their advice."

In the time that has passed since he wrote these statements, the distinctions between what an informal system will and will not do have become somewhat blurred. Where does one place a medical site that offers diagnostic conclusions and treatment rec-ommendations online without ever seeing the patient? This kind of site appears in some ways to be a formal information system. Yet, it functions outside the scope or model of what generally is considered to be appropriate professional practice. How can the user evaluate the quality of information provided at this site if it is no longer bound by the formal models of the profession?

Similar—though perhaps not quite so dramatic—questions can be raised about many information systems that clearly are informal. Consider the following example:

A patient who is experiencing continued, severe pain at the surgical site of a cardiac triple bypass procedure is becoming increasingly distressed by his condition. The pain is sufficiently severe that wearing clothing over the incision site remains ex-tremely uncomfortable. His cardiologist tells him that the pain is a result of the use of retractors during surgery, which pull back the rib cage to provide access to the heart. Application of re-tractors disturbs both bones and muscles, resulting in residual sensitivity for at least several months. The patient has consid-ered his physician's information and concludes that the pain is more than "sensitivity" and has lasted more than "several" months. He wants to know how other bypass patients experi-ence the aftermath of their surgeries, in order to try to place his own symptoms within the range of what is a "normal" versus an "abnormal" response.

Access to the Internet permits the twenty-first century pa-tient to gather information that bears on his question through a number of venues. Two of the primary options open to him are to post his question on a Web site bulletin board devoted to health or surgical or cardiac issues, or find a relevant chat room and query its members. Suppose he takes the first option, post-ing his question on a cardiac surgery bulletin board. Rapidly, he receives a series of responses. Depending on who is online at the time, who is attracted to the particular bulletin board, and quite a number of other circumstances beyond the user's knowledge, the responses he receives can be quite different. For example, he might post his query late at night, when he is having difficulty sleeping because of his pain. The responses he receives are from individuals who also report a great deal of pain for a long time after surgery. Should the user conclude, based on this informal system of gathering information, that his pain is the norm, something all post-bypass patients must live with? Or, is it possible that the responses have come from a select group of post-bypass patients who, like himself, cannot sleep due to their pain and are, therefore, spending late hours online?

Other scenarios could be generated that would lead to the reverse conclusion: that the user's pain is very atypical, something about which to be concerned, and a point which should lead him to question seriously his physician's expertise. A third possibility is that the patient will receive no responses to his query. How should he interpret this lack of communication? Does it mean that there is "no one out there with a similar problem" signifying that he truly is experiencing something bizarre and atypical? Or does the lack of response mean simply that he has tapped the wrong site to get to the people who might be in a position similar to his own? Finally, his query might elicit what could be considered irrelevant information. For example, he might receive emotionally targeted responses, such as sympathy for his pain or criticism of his expectations of surgical recovery. He also might receive responses from Internet "pretenders," individuals who fabricate responses or identities, using the informal system to role-play anyone they please for a wide range of usually unhelpful reasons.

Given the problems that can arise when using informal information systems on the Internet, it is helpful to have a set of questions in mind to assist in evaluating the material that is being retrieved and the retrieval mechanism that has been used. Following are three general questions that can be applied when using informal information systems on the Internet:

1. *What kinds of "errors" in sampling might have occurred?* Since all responses to posted queries are by what is called self-selection, how might the respondees have selected to

communicate? Is there some glaring bias in the set of respondees, such as those who are sleepless across the U.S.
time zones due to pain and, therefore, available to respond to a midnight query? Also in this category, does the
site itself tap a biased sample? For instance, an alternative
medicine bulletin board might be more likely than a traditional medicine bulletin board to draw individuals who
have responded poorly to traditional treatments.

2. *When are threats to credibility most problematic?* Here is
the issue: anyone—a "pretender" of any ilk, a 7-year old
child who has just gotten access to the family computer—
can respond to most posted queries. If the user can be
comfortable with the range of bizarre and useless responses that may be retrieved, and has a way to separate
them from the helpful responses, these are steps in the
right direction. Problems arise when what the user really
needs is the kind of information best obtained from formal
information systems, or from known experts, but seeks
answers informally instead. If the user endows these informal answers with the same credibility that would be given
to formal information, the user could be in for trouble.

3. *How important is accountability?* Accountability involves assuming responsibility for one's actions. Com-
municators on the informal information sectors of the
Internet are only very rarely held accountable for what
they say or do. In general, no system of accountability
exists in the informal systems. If the user wants an answer to an important question that will impact his medical treatment, and he seeks this answer informally, he
places himself in the vulnerable position of listening to
others who bear no responsibility for their actions—even
if those actions are deliberate efforts to sabotage treatment. On the other hand, if he wants someone to talk
with about his experiences or is attempting to deal with
issues of loneliness or isolation, the benefits he might
obtain from informal systems can outweigh issues of accountability. As with credibility, it is when users are unclear about the distinction between informal and formal

information systems or, for some reason, choose one when they would be best advised to choose the other, problems are more likely to arise.

Suggested References .....

Coiera, E. (1997). *Guide to medical informatics, the Internet and telemedicine*. New York: Chapman & Hall Medical. This ancillary text proceeds from an introduction to basic concepts in informatics, through types of information systems in health care, to a thorough discussion of the Internet from a medical perspective. The book is unique in its use of models rather than Web-based examples. This orientation gives it a timeless quality that will prove useful to readers who would like to pursue topics such as medical information systems in more depth.

Denzin, N. K., & Lincoln, Y. S., Eds. (2000). *Handbook of qualitative research (2nd Ed.)*. Thousand Oaks, CA: Sage Publications, Inc. This is a huge, edited volume that is appropriate for readers who would like more familiarity with qualitative types of information and the philosophies that have shaped the research processes of contextualization and deconstruction in the social sciences. It contains works by dozens of authors whose writing spans the history, paradigms, methods, and interpretations of qualitative material.

Ferguson, T. (1996). *Health online*. Reading, MA: Addison-Wesley Publishing Company. This is a how-to book for users of medical information in cyberspace. It provides hand holding for beginning use of e-mail as well as Web surfing, and provides a good perspective on what is available on the Internet. While some of the material is by now dated, the general orientation of the book and the categories of Internet sources described remain quite useful.

Citations in Text .....

Bereners-Lee, T., Calliau, R., Loutonen, A., & Nielsen, H. F. (1994). A secret, the World Wide Web. *Communications of the ACM 37*(8), 76–82.

Clancy, W. J. (1995). In L. Steels & R. Brooks (Eds.), *The artificial life route to artificial intelligence*. New Jersey: Lawrence Erlbaum.

Clough, P. T. (1998). *The ends of ethnography: From realism to social criticism (2nd Ed.)*. New York: Peter Lang.

Coiera, E. (See Suggested References.)

Derrida, J. (1976). *Of grammatology*. (G. C. Spivak, Trans.). Baltimore: Johns Hopkins University Press.

Ferguson, T. (See Suggested References.)

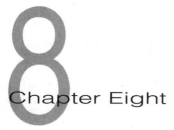

Chapter Eight

Artificial Intelligence in Medical Informatics

> The emergence of machine intelligence during the second half of the twentieth century is the most important development in the evolution of this planet since the origin of life two to three thousand million years ago.
>
> T. Stonier

Introduction

The above quote is a powerful assessment of the promise of artificial intelligence (AI), particularly since the most common question still asked about AI is, "What is it?" Answering this question is difficult for AI experts as well as for nonexperts who find themselves increasingly confronted with reports of AI techniques in the medical literature. Conferences of internationally known AI experts have been convened solely to define the realm of AI and to project its possible impact on society.

Many health care providers perceive AI as just another set of computer-based tools touted by some as the brilliant answer to medical questions. When health care providers ask, "What is AI?" they typically mean, "What makes AI different from the mathematical modeling, complex statistical techniques, and formal decision analyses that have been appearing in the medical literature for quite a few years?"

Following are a few points that may help in the struggle to grasp the meaning and importance of AI:

1. AI is not one single approach or program (see later section on Types of Expert Systems), but rather a collection of different approaches aimed at the general goal of getting computers to perform "cognitive" tasks that had been believed previously to be the exclusive realm of the human brain.

2. One of the most fundamental goals of AI has been the development of what is termed "expert systems." Expert systems are computer programs designed to perform tasks as well as or better than human experts. In medicine, expert diagnostic systems have been developed to perform such tasks as diagnosing infectious diseases and recommending treatments for them (i.e., the expert system known as MYCIN).

3. AI differs from other computerized medical systems in a very important way: Instead of performing the computational tasks of a glorified calculator, as is the case with many computer programs, AI refers to computer-based systems that are capable of reasoning, finding problems, thinking, or making inferences.

4. Because AI systems are expected to be reasoning machines, they have held out the vast promise of performing better than human experts at such tasks as making medical diagnoses. One of the fundamental reasons that machines might prove superior to humans on some tasks is because the human mind, even the mind of the expert, becomes overwhelmed by the explosion of information and cannot cope with the number of pieces of information that must be taken into account simultaneously to arrive at the best possible conclusions/solutions.

The next two questions typically asked about AI systems are: "Do they work?" and "How do they work?" Before answering these questions, some background information on AI and expert systems is in order.

A Brief History of Artificial Intelligence ....

■THE ORIGINS OF AI

Many individuals who are not AI scientists are surprised to learn that AI has been in existence since the middle of the twentieth century. (And the history of the idea of AI can be traced back to the ancient Greek philosophers!)

The AI of the last half of the twentieth century appears to have grown out of the need for "machines" that could handle other kinds of information besides numerical calculations. If you recall the discussion of ENIAC in Chapter 1, the first machine recognized as a true computer, you will remember that its functions were limited to high speed addition and multiplication. Even with the advent of programming languages (remember, the first computers did not operate through software programs but rather via a system of switches), the basic functions of computers remained mathematical in nature. The early programming languages that were developed, such as FORTRAN, were designed to facilitate the programming of mathematical functions, such as high level algebra.

Today, when "software" literally is a household term, it is almost incomprehensible that computers once operated without software. And that the "user-friendly" software in abundance today is based on high level programming languages about which the user need know absolutely nothing!

Stepping back into computer history, we see that individuals in many sciences began to wish for machines that could do more than mathematics. In 1956, a meeting was held at Dartmouth College for researchers who were interested in the potential for computers to act as "reasoning" machines. It was at this meeting that John McCarthy coined the term "artificial intelligence" to refer to the possibilities envisioned for computer usage.

In the ensuing years, it became clear that AI scientists tended toward one of two camps in their research and development efforts. Some scientists set as their goal replication of the functioning of the human mind. For these scientists, the most important achievement is to produce computers that "think" like humans, even if the thinking tasks are very small and insignificant in themselves, such as building a computer robot that can put one wooden block on top of another. Many individuals in this camp are cognitive scientists whose primary interest is understanding human thinking through the development of computer systems that mimic it. Other scientists focus on computer systems that produce correct answers to problems, regardless of whether the computer arrives at the answers the way a human would or not. In other words, this second group of scientists tends to be more focused on the practical usefulness of AI rather than its use in advancing the understanding of human cognition. Medical AI falls primarily into this second camp, since its most important function has been to act as a consultant to physicians.

■THE EMERGENCE OF EXPERT SYSTEMS

During the late 1960s and the 1970s, AI research took a turn toward the development of commercially viable programs, i.e., programs that could compete or even surpass experts in the ability to solve nonmathematical problems. The origin of expert systems was not in medicine, but rather in the "hard" sciences, with the success of DENDRAL, a program commissioned by NASA to perform analysis of chemical structures on board spacecraft.

DENDRAL served as a prototype for expert systems in other areas—for DENDRAL was, in every sense, an expert in the field of mass-spectrogram analysis. DENDRAL's knowledge base had been gleaned from human experts in this subfield of chemistry. (For a detailed retrospective on the development and applications of DENDRAL see Lindsay et al., 1980.)

Using DENDRAL's pioneering approach of "capturing" the knowledge of human experts and incorporating it into computer programs, the Stanford University group that built DENDRAL proceeded to build the first viable expert system in medicine. It was named MYCIN (Shortliffe, 1976; Buchanan & Shortliffe, 1984), and its purposes were to diagnose infectious diseases and to prescribe appropriate treatments. In short, MYCIN was intended to act as a consultant to physicians in a very specific, very clear area of clinical medicine. Of course, MYCIN needed a knowledge base in its specialty area, a task undertaken by professionals that have come to be known as knowledge engineers (Feigenbaum, 1980). MYCIN's knowledge engineers worked with medical experts in infectious diseases to lay out the knowledge base that would be programmed into MYCIN as a set of rules (see later discussion on rule-based systems).

Remember, however, that medical reasoning often is done under conditions of uncertainty (refer to Chapter 2 on the Nature of Medical Reasoning and the Limits of Medical Information). Frequently, even the best of experts in a field might not have adequate information or might have conflicting information about a case, which means that a diagnostic and/or treatment decision must be made with some degree of uncertainty. Consequently, medical expert systems also must be capable of operating under conditions of uncertainty. This means that the rules human experts provide for a computerized expert system are not enough. Said another way, an expert system must consist not only of a knowledge base, but also of some way of making inferences from the knowledge base under conditions of uncertainty. This mechanism for making inferences is commonly called an inference engine. In simple terms, it is the part of the computer's expert system that makes the best guess about a diagnosis or treatment in the face of imperfect information.

On the heels of the relatively successful MYCIN, another group of researchers built INTERNIST (Pople et al., 1975). INTERNIST attempted to capture all the knowledge available in internal medicine, including its subspecialty areas, and initially included approximately 100,000 "rules." INTERNIST has undergone a number of revisions, but has had limited success, probably due to the attempt to capture all of internal medicine in a cumbersome series of rules.

In the nonmedical domain, AI scientists had already begun to recognize that true experts in any field do not grind through hundreds of thousands of "rules" before making a decision. One of the central demonstrations of this fact was done on research with the game of chess. A series of experiments with chess masters versus novices (de Groot, 1965, 1966) had shown that the chess master considered fewer moves than the novice and seemed to think about chess in terms of entire board positions rather than the positions of individual chess pieces. (See Fig. 8a.)

From this and similar, subsequent research, it has become clear that experts "distill" their knowledge in some way. They formulate the problem at hand in a very different manner than do novices, who do not have the cognitive "shortcuts" present in experts.

As a result of such findings, other approaches to expert systems have been developed. While a knowledge base remains essential, as does a way to make inferences, i.e., an inference engine, programming is no longer limited to the single approach of listing what may seem an interminable number of rules. Rule-based expert systems are contrasted with other approaches to medical expert systems in the discussions that follow.

Usefulness of Medical Expert Systems

After "What is AI?" the second question most health care providers ask about AI systems is, "Do they work?"

To understand the answer, begin with an awareness of the fact that the future of AI is uncertain. While the computer world has experienced frustration in the development of commercially useful AI systems in complex fields such as medicine, the answer is not clearly "yes" or "no." Machines that think and learn can, and have been, developed. ("Machine" in this context, refers to both software programs and computer hardware.) However, capturing the knowledge necessary to produce "expert level" performance is a major hurdle, as is the practical problem of keeping a machine's knowledge base up to date in a

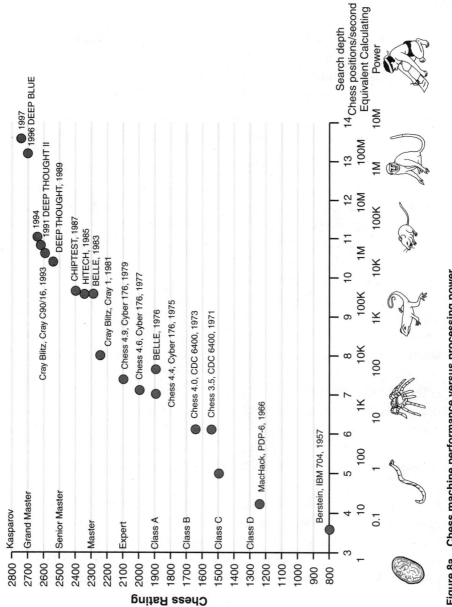

Figure 8a   Chess machine performance versus processing power.

field such as medicine, which is undergoing a continuing information explosion.

To better understand why AI systems in medicine, i.e., medical expert systems, fail to work as effectively as is theoretically possible, consider the following example:

You are an "expert" driver, an individual who has been driving a car nearly every day for more than 10 years. You are an expert in the sense that driving has become "second nature" to you, i.e., you perform the necessary tasks rather automatically, without having to think them through, step by step. In fact, you can carry on a conversation while you are driving, or listen to the morning news on your car radio. Now, think about how you would go about teaching someone to drive who has never driven before. What would you do?

If you actually have been driving for quite some time, and you are not a driving instructor, you would probably experience some difficulty teaching a true novice what to do behind the wheel. Would it occur to you to tell your "student" that the key must be turned in the ignition before anything else can happen? (Many computer instructors in past years have made the analogous mistake of failing to tell their students to turn on the computer!) Would you remember to tell your student driver to be sure the transmission is in "park" before turning on the ignition? How would you convey the "feel" of the gas and break pedals, i.e., using just the right amount of foot pressure to move forward and to stop. How would you convey the sense of time and distance, as in judging whether you have adequate time to make a turn against traffic with other vehicles approaching at a busy intersection? Yes, the laws of physics apply, but these laws are not what you, the expert driver, use in mathematical calculations to make your decision to cut out or to wait. In short, how do you convey your complex knowledge/skill base, developed from much experience, to the abject beginner?

A similar problem occurs when AI experts attempt to "capture" the knowledge of expert physicians in order to develop computerized expert systems. Expert physicians know a great deal that they can express in words, but they also "know" a great deal that they do not express. Like the expert driver, so much has become "second nature" that the steps that once led them to their conclusions, or which guided their thinking, seem to have evaporated. Some cognitive scientists believe that as an individual progresses from novice to expert, the "rules" or "steps" which initially guided their cognitions degrade. This means that the small steps that once were necessary to make a diagnosis are no longer necessary, and the expert "jumps" to a working diagnosis without awareness of preliminary reasoning. This is analogous to the chess master who thinks in terms of an entire board instead of individual chess pieces.

Consider this simple case: An expert physician walks into a hospital room to see a patient she has never before evaluated. The physician enters the room, takes a glance at the patient, lifts the sheet to palpate one side of the abdomen very quickly, and immediately orders a range of liver function tests and imaging studies, having made a working diagnosis of liver disease. The patient may be appalled by the rapidity with which the initial diagnosis was made, and the accompanying third-year medical students are amazed. If the medical students were to ask the expert how she arrived at her immediate, working diagnosis, she may have to struggle to put herself back in the place of a novice. She may be successful enough at doing this to state some of the "rules" to her students: The patient's room had an odor of ammonia, typical of advanced hepatic disease in which the liver fails to clear nitrogenous wastes and other toxic substances properly from the blood, ergo the smell. Second, the patient's skin was too yellow for a Caucasian, jaundiced in fact, and the discoloration was even visible in the patient's eyes. Palpation of the liver confirmed enlargement. Thus, the expert has transmitted some of her rules to her students. However, the expert physician did not actually go through these rules, step-by-step, in her own head. Instead, she was "hit" by a gestalt, a total olfactory, visual, and tactile picture which said to her "liver disease." The point is that transmitting the rules does not add up to a model of how the expert physician thinks about the case or arrives at a working diagnosis.

Return for a moment to philosophy of science. Polanyi (1972) noted that, "By watching the master . . . the apprentice unconsciously picks up the rules of the art, including those which are not explicitly known to the master himself." What Polanyi meant by this statement is not that the expert was ignorant in the acquisition of his/her knowledge, but rather that there is more to expertise than the expert can readily articulate because he or she has progressed far from the point at which every small step must be thought through, and has entered the realm of "second nature" performance. Interestingly, this apprenticeship model is precisely what Flexner promoted in his discussion of medical learning through bedside rounds more than 50 years before! (See Chapter 1.)

Interviews and in-depth questioning of medical experts to capture a knowledge base has not led successfully to expert systems—instead, it appears more feasible to build "novice" systems comprised of step-by-step knowledge. Of course, this is not the intent of those researchers who have tried to develop expert systems.

In a provocative conclusion to a paper on cognitive issues in AI, Dreyfus (1979) made the statement that AI experts have long believed the Socratic slogan that, "If you understand it, you can explain it." Dreyfus suggested that in the case of expert systems the slogan should be reversed, "Anyone who thinks he can fully explain his skill does not have expert understanding."

How Medical Expert Systems Work

■TYPES OF EXPERT SYSTEMS

Perhaps the third question most commonly raised by individuals who have made it through the "what is it" and "does it work" stages, is "How does AI work, even when it works imperfectly?"

There are several answers to this third question because AI is a collection of techniques and approaches. This section discusses three approaches to AI expert systems that are commonly used in medical applications: rule-based systems, frame-based systems, and neural networks.

Rule-Based Systems

Of the three approaches to AI discussed in this chapter, rule-based systems tend to be the easiest to grasp because they do not depart all that dramatically from conventional computer programming. You do not need to be a computer programmer to comprehend the fundamental characteristics of rule-based systems, but if you have done some programming you will see similarities.

Rule-based systems are precisely what the name implies: They are expert systems (computer programs) that contain a series of logical rules, often a very long list of rules. In medicine, the rules contained in a rule-based system pertain to diagnosis or treatment of diseases.

The creation of INTERNIST, the pioneering effort to cover all of internal medicine in a rule-based system, is a good example from which to learn about how rule-based systems work. The "expert" in this case was the medical internist who worked on the system. In order to make a diagnosis, INTERNIST requires the user to enter the signs and symptoms presented by the patient. Let us suppose that a patient comes to see his physician because he is experiencing some difficulty breathing. INTERNIST will want some additional information about the patient, similar to that contained in a typical history and physical exam. Included in this information might be the age of the patient, his height and weight, whether he has a fever, any history of cardiac or pulmonary disease, or any allergies. INTERNIST may also require information about the kind of breathing problem the patient is experiencing: Is it shortness of breath? Does he wheeze? Is the breathing problem constant or intermittent? If intermittent, when is it most likely to occur? Did the patient have a chest X-ray taken? If so, is the film normal or abnormal? Has the patient recently been in contact with anyone known to have tuberculosis? Is the patient's tuberculin skin test normal?

This input to the computer will be churned through a long list of "rules." Here is a simplified version of what the kinds of logical rules in a rule-based expert system might be:

- If this patient does not have a fever, he probably does not have an active respiratory infection.
- If his chest X-ray is normal, he probably does not have pneumonia. This, added to the absence of fever, strengthens the hypothesis that he does not have an active infection.
- If his tuberculin skin test is negative, he probably is not infected with TB. The normal chest X-ray strengthens the hypothesis that he does not have an active TB infection.
- He has no history of cardiac or pulmonary disease, and no previous allergies.
- This helps suggest that he is not suffering from heart disease, although a cardiac work-up might be suggested in order to avoid the slight chance of a very serious problem.
- The patient reports that his breathing problem is intermittent: It occurs after exercise. He also reports that the nature of his problem is wheezing and shortness of breath. These facts suggest a pulmonary problem brought on by exercise. The wheezing nature of the problem is most characteristic of asthma.
- Most likely diagnostic conclusion from the information provided:
  exercised-induced asthma

When a rule-based expert system actually runs the data on a patient case, it churns through many more rules than the selected ones above. For the sake of the example, the rules have been limited to those that are most relevant and salient, and they have been translated completely into English. In reality, the rule-based expert system would test many more rules, many of which would be totally irrelevant, such as whether the patient has blood in his stool, or whether he is experiencing circulatory problems in his hands and feet. Such a system may contain hundreds or thousands of rules, all of which would be applied to each case. The ones that are "diagnostic" in this case are probably the normal X-ray, lack of fever, and especially the wheezing after exercise. In short, rule-based systems are cumbersome in many ways: They are inefficient because they have no way early on to separate irrelevant from relevant information and must therefore "test" every possible rule for every case.

Rule-based expert systems can indicate the degree of certainty with which the diagnosis is made, and can suggest the need for further information such as additional medical tests, in order to provide greater certainty of diagnosis. Such systems can also be "tailored" to fit the patient population at a particular health care site or geographic location. For example, at a site in which HIV disease is highly prevalent, there is a higher probability that a patient with breathing problems, even with a negative tuberculin test, might have TB. Consequently, the certainty or probability with which the diagnosis of exercised-induced asthma can be made will be lower, and other relevant tests might be required in order to rule out other, more serious problems.

Frame-Based Systems

There is no perfect heading for this category of expert systems because "frame" is only one of several terms and approaches that have been used to label a movement toward a different way of representing knowledge.

Rule-based expert systems are problematic, not only because it takes time for them to churn through all rules for every case, but also for two additional reasons:

1. If something needs to be reprogrammed, the job is massive if it is doable at all. Consider that the initial version of INTERNIST contained over 100,000 logical rules. Also consider that it was developed before the discovery of HIV disease. Now, all signs and symptoms that may

suggest HIV/AIDS must be included in an expert diagnostic system. Think about the job of going through
every one of 100,000 rules to see if it is connected with
a possible diagnosis of HIV disease!

2. Cognitive research had begun to suggest that experts
(as the chess masters) do not think in terms of step-by-
step rules. Instead, experts appear to "chunk" their
knowledge together (as in the earlier example of the
physician who made a working diagnosis of liver disease
based on a gestalt of information rather than individual
pieces of data.) Minsky (1975) was one of the first computer scientists to suggest that knowledge in an expert
system should be represented in chunks rather than in
individual rules.

A helpful way to think about expert systems that use chunked knowledge is to consider that the knowledge is entered into
the system in a kind of "pattern." Whether the pattern is called
a frame or a script or some other term used by a given group of
scientists, the important point is that knowledge that fits together is put into the computer's knowledge base together.

If knowledge about HIV disease were to be programmed
into a computer's knowledge base as a pattern, such signs and
symptoms as fever of unknown origin, unexplained weight loss,
lymphadenopathy, and history of intravenous drug use might
be chunked, or "framed" together. Information that relates to
HIV disease is clustered together, while information irrelevant to
HIV is excluded from this frame.

One practical benefit of this kind of expert system is that it
is easier to reprogram than a rule-based system. For example,
as CD4 cell counts and viral load began to be used in the diagnosis of HIV disease, as well as to index disease severity, the
"frame" for HIV disease could be reprogrammed to include information on CD4 cells and viral loads without touching the
frames for unrelated diseases, such as breast cancer.

Another advantage of chunking knowledge is that this approach appears to reflect how experts think more closely than do

rule-based systems that do not use chunked knowledge. Consequently, this approach may provide a better route to the development of expert systems that truly function like human experts. Please note, however, that medical expert systems that use some form of chunked knowledge have been developed typically for their practical value, rather than their value for understanding human cognition. While these systems may, as an offshoot, teach us something about how human cognition actually works, their major role has been to provide useful, "second-opinion" tools and teaching devices. An example of this type of system is ILIAD (Warner et al., 1988), which is still in use as a prototype teaching tool and can be tailored to the patient population at particular sites through the use of a special "authoring kit."

Neural Networks

Of the three kinds of expert systems discussed in this chapter, neural networks have grown most clearly out of a desire to understand and mimic the human cognitive apparatus. Even the name, "neural" networks speaks of an inclination to make the electronic machine mimic the biological one.

To grasp the essence of the neural network, think back to what we believe we know about the human brain. The brain is comprised of billions of neurons that communicate with each other through connections. When connections are damaged, as in a stroke, the neurological linkages that make normal behavior possible are disrupted, i.e., a stroke in the speech center of the brain may deprive the patient of her ability to use words to express thoughts and emotions.

Now, think about the other side of the coin: how human speech is learned. Given that the muscles of a child's oral pharynx and larynx are at an appropriate level of development, speech is acquired through a process of "training" the appropriate neurological connections that result in organized vocalizations. While this is a simplification of an exquisitely complex and refined neuromuscular process, what is crucial to this example is the issue of "training." By training, in this instance, we mean a process of input (hearing spoken language), production (experimenting with phonation), and feedback (refinement through correction or validation).

Neural networks are designed to function in a similar manner, albeit via computer circuitry rather than human neurons. Computerized neural networks are "trained" by association. Data are input into the neural network, data about which correct responses are already known. Lawrence (1991, p. 5) provides a simple example of how a computerized neural network can be trained to recognize vegetables from their descriptions:

> Let's suppose our untrained network initially decides that a large, round, orange vegetable is a zucchini. The training example, which has the correct output, says the vegetable is actually a pumpkin. The neural network simulation software looks at the correct output and realizes that its guess was wrong. The software then makes changes to its internal connections so that the next time it sees the same inputs, it will be more likely to produce the correct answer. The connections are adjusted so that the inputs are associated more strongly with the pumpkin output and less strongly with the zucchini output. This training is repeated for a set of examples until the network learns the correct answers.

Now, consider the use of a computerized neural network in medicine. A recent problem that has troubled clinicians working with HIV patients is the difficulty of making accurate prognoses regarding life expectancies. This problem has eluded traditional statistical models probably because we have insufficient insight into the roles of specific variables in predicting mortality. On the other hand, sufficient data have now been gathered regarding the clinical course of a substantial sample of patients, as well as their actual life spans. When these data were used to train a computerized neural network (Montgomery et al., 1995), the network was able to train to an unanticipated degree of accuracy, i.e., approximately 95%. What the network "learned" is not "visible" to the researchers (just as the biological connections in the brain are not transparent even to the expert neurologist). However, the adjustments the computerized system made to its own connections permitted a great deal of accuracy in predicting life expectancy outcomes; and it can be used to help physicians generate prognoses.

While many neural networks are in use primarily for the study of cognition, others have begun to prove themselves useful in helping solve practical problems.

■SOME CAVEATS

While it is true that the development of expert systems has met with a degree of disappointment since the golden promises of the early years, a number of satisfactory expert systems are in use today. Departing from medicine for a moment, consider the fact that "expert systems" are used to diagnose car problems at some dealerships. These may not be highly sophisticated expert systems, but they do incorporate some expert system concepts in a practical and relatively cost-effective manner. In medicine, expert systems are in use presently in a number of areas, including EKG Interpreters, Pap smear screenings as in PAPNET, and in antibiotic decision support.

Weiss and Kulikowski (1991) have proposed that a strict adherence to AI "expert systems" be abandoned in favor of "computer systems that learn" using many kinds of functions, including true AI as well as statistical models. AI arose initially in response to the need to manage information that was not primarily mathematical. What Weiss and Kulikowski have called for is a combination of mathematical and nonmathematical approaches that may provide us with the best of both worlds. They state that, "A *learning system* is a computer program that makes decisions based on the accumulated experience contained in successfully solved cases. Unlike an *expert system*, which solves problems using a computer model of expert human reasoning, a pure learning system can use many different techniques for exploiting the computational power of a computer, regardless of their relation to human cognitive processes." Clearly, these scientists are suggesting that a practical approach be taken to AI, even including statistics, in order to get the most useful output without rigidly adhering to earlier definitions of expert systems.

This combined approach is practical: Its goal is to deal with complex, real-world problems and to use whatever techniques are available to arrive at correct judgments or solutions.

When considering whether to invest time in learning how to use an expert system or a learning system, consider whether the system will provide practical results. Bear in mind the position taken above: If your interest is in getting the best medical advice possible regardless of the AI approach used to obtain it, avoid getting caught up in one "camp" versus another. For example, if you are practicing in a geographic area in which there are no experts in treating infection, the Computer-Assisted Management Program for Antibiotics and Other Antiinfective Agents developed by Evans, et al (1998) might help you decide on a treatment plan. Worrying about whether it is rule-based, frame-based, or a form of neural network might be quite irrelevant to your purposes. And if you have at your disposal a system that is partly statistical and partly nonmathematical AI, and it works well, use it! Additional hints for the use of AI in medicine follow.

Using Artificial Intelligence Intelligently ....

■HINTS FOR USING EXPERT AND LEARNING SYSTEMS

Here are some points to help you decide whether a particular expert system or learning system is worth exploring:

1. Decide on your priorities. If what you need is a practical system to help you make emergency decisions in the absence of top-notch experts, look for systems that have a very high "hit rate," i.e., systems that do as well as good physicians.
2. Learn how to find out about the practical usefulness of systems in your area. Some medical journals, such as

the *New England Journal of Medicine*, have regularly published comparisons between judgments made by good expert systems versus those made by practicing physicians.

3. Be aware of the crucial distinction between systems developed with the primary goal of achieving the best artificial "advice" possible, versus those that have been developed primarily to attempt to mirror the workings of the human mind. If you are a cognitive scientist, you may be interested in the latter. Otherwise, you are probably best advised to focus on the former.

4. Get familiar with where your AI system's "blind spots" are. What kinds of medical problems does it have difficulty identifying correctly? Or, in which therapeutic domains is it especially weak? What kinds of mistakes does it commonly make (and should you watch out for)? On the other hand, in which types of situations does it have a track record for outperforming human experts?

■WORKING WITH AN AI TYPE SYSTEM

Availability

Until the past few years, computer-based systems for making medical diagnoses and treatment suggestions were not easily accessible:

1. Many were in prototype form, meaning that they were being tested at selected sites and not ready for commercial distribution. It can be extremely difficult to gain access to such systems when they are still under development.

2. Many were running on larger computers than were available to most individuals and health care sites. For example, they were often developed to run initially on AI work stations rather than on personal computers or even high powered minicomputers.

3. Authoring kits for the systems were not readily available. What this means, for example, is that if the prevalence of HIV in Utah where ILIAD was developed is far lower than the prevalence of HIV at the urban health center where you work, you could not change the likelihood that a patient who presented at your site with fever of unknown origin, unexplained weight loss, and history of intravenous drug use might have HIV disease.

4. Finally, the existing programs have not been "user friendly." Not only did some of them require extensive training in order to get to first base, but most required the level of medical knowledge expected at the M.D. or post-graduate, subspecialty level. Such systems demanded so much of their users that their "audience" was relatively narrow. The systems were designed to query the user at various points, and if the user did not possess adequate knowledge to respond to the system, everything would grind to a halt.

Many of the above issues are changing. Systems are now being built for typical, desktop computers; user-friendliness is increasing; and authoring systems are being developed. On the downside, most systems available for desktop use are not powerful diagnostic systems; they are more akin to computerized medical encyclopedias.

■RUNNING THE SYSTEM

If you have the opportunity to access an expert system or learning system that addresses your needs, you should expect to do the following:

1. Run a broad range of test cases. Compare the computer's responses with those of physicians whose expertise in the particular areas is solid. Then try to reconcile any differences.

2. Compare crucial estimates used in the system. Get an authoring kit to make changes when the estimates do

not fit your site. For example, if the expert system you are using sets the prevalence of TB at 8%, but in your hospital's community, the prevalence is 20%, this must be changed to make the system as accurate as possible at your site.

3. Recognize the importance of site-specific and time-specific differences. For example, if an expert system was developed before the emergence of HIV disease, or when knowledge of the disease was embryonic, it would need adjustments to provide optimal output, particularly at sites where the prevalence of HIV disease is high.

4. Determine what kind of assistance you need to input your cases as well as to interpret your output. Note that many systems will query you about the case you are investigating, so if you are not a physician, you will want to ask a physician colleague who is familiar with the case to assist you on the clinical "interactions" aspect. For example, if results of a biopsy were not entered for a particular patient with a suspicious bone lesion, the program may request biopsy data. Perhaps attempts at biopsy were unsuccessful in obtaining good samples because the patient had undergone radiation treatments to the area. Without knowing about the relation between radiation and biopsy information, you might get stuck in running the system, which is likely to continue to request biopsy information until it "understands" the history of radiation.

5. Check for areas in which the system is good and those in which it does poorly. Rarely is an expert system equally strong in all areas of medicine since it will typically reflect the expertise of those who have developed it. Find out whether the developers were infectious disease experts, cardiologists, hematologists, pulmonologists, etc. Try to use the system for the kinds of cases in which it is likely to be strongest—but remember that a strength in one area coupled with weaknesses in other areas of medicine can come up with weak conclusions.

For example, a system strong in diagnosing respiratory diseases might overlook a relatively rare but life-threatening cardiac cause of respiratory distress.

6. At this stage in the development of AI and learning systems, do not rely solely on the system to direct your treatment or diagnostic plans! Instead, use the printout as a kind of second opinion, or as a check on what you have come up with. Perhaps you have missed something that the system can identify. On the other hand, the system may very likely have missed something particular to your site or patient. Remember that since expert systems are created by humans, they are likely to be characterized by human biases. Even expert systems that learn are likely to learn in the ways their creators decided to equip them.

Finally, The Future

Given the successes as well as the failures of artificial intelligence in medical applications, what are we likely to see in the foreseeable future? Another way to ask this question is, given the technologies that are in place now in prototype form, what can we realistically expect to see within the next 5 to 10 years?

One of the most promising and practical avenues for artificial intelligence applications are attempts to improve patient information, such as the prototype called "Guardian Angel." In such systems, a huge database on a sample of one (i.e., a single patient) is encoded on a card the size of a credit card. When the patient seeks consultation or treatment, the patient database card is scanned to see if there are any red flags, that is, any possibilities of increased risk based on medication interactions, co-existing medical conditions, other medical history information. Using such a system bypasses the limitations of human memory, self-report data, and the problems of finding hospital or clinic charts.

Are there ethical ramifications of such systems? In other words, does the patient have the right to keep private any of his/her health information by withholding it from the physician? Suppose a woman was diagnosed as schizophrenic at age 16. After a week of hospitalization, symptoms remitted, leaving the patient functioning normally until her present age of 45 years. Now she is seeking physician assistance for chronic pain that appears to be related to arthritis, but which seems to be excessively severe given the arthritic changes seen on imaging studies. The patient is concerned that if the physician notes a psychiatric history, he or she will not take her pain problem seriously and might relegate it to a psychosomatic problem. Knowing what we know about bias in medical decision making, the patient could be correct in assuming that her psychiatric history might impact negatively on the extensiveness of her pain work-up and her treatment with analgesic medications.

Now consider a dramatically different situation. A patient visits her physician for what appears to be a recurrence of bronchitis. As a result of coughing, she is experiencing chest pain. Because the woman has had a history of intermittently abnormal electrocardiograms, the physician decides to treat her with a vasodilator as well as medication for the bronchitis. The point of the vasodilator is to help ensure that the workload on the patient's heart will not trigger a heart attack until she can be brought into the hospital for a more extensive cardiac work up. The patient fails to tell her physician that she is hypotensive, and because she is anxious about her respiratory problem as well as her chest pain, her blood pressure rises to normal levels when taken in the physician's office. This patient did not want to withhold information about hypotension from her physician— she simply did not know it was important. After taking the vasodilator for 3 days, her hypotension fell to extreme levels. She lost consciousness, suffered a concussion as she fell to the floor, and ultimately escaped more severe consequences when she was found by a friend who phoned the local first-aid squad. There also may be situations in which patients forget or are unaware of a diagnosis made earlier that impinges on today's medical treatment decision. For example, perhaps a patient with a urinary tract infection (UTI) seeks treatment, and the treating physician prescribes Bactrim, which is appropriate in the vast majority of cases. But the patient has a genetic condition called G6PD deficiency that was diagnosed in childhood, which she has little knowledge about. She has no reason to reflect on this when she presents her current problem to her physician. Because of her condition, treating her UTI with Bactrim could cause life-threatening hemolytic anemia. Use of something like the Guardian Angel in this case could save a life.

The new AI applications also provide other services to the physician, one of which is "learning" about the kinds of information the health care provider typically seeks in patient records, as well as the order in which the information is sought (thus, reflecting the thinking process of the individual medical expert). These applications could make the health care provider's job far more efficient. Cardiologists would probably be alerted first to any history of coronary artery disease, as well as family history of heart problems. Dentists, on the other hand, would probably be provided cardiac information early in the information search primarily if the patient had risk factors for endocarditis, which could require medication with antibiotics for dental procedures. The priorities given to particular kinds of information would be based on what the system had already learned about the priorities of the health care provider using the system. This process differs dramatically from the health care provider going through a full history on each patient, a process that can bring into view factors which might not be typical for that health care provider to seek, but which might be important for diagnostic and treatment decisions. For example, since hypertension is a much more common problem than hypotension in Western cultures, the physician who added vasodilators to the bronchitis patient's regimen might have taught her system to provide red flags only for hypertension. If this were the case, using such a system would not have helped her to know about her patient's history of hypotension, even if the information had been entered into the patient's database and scanned by the physician's "information assistant" program.

In short, our immediate future appears to hold out the promise of better information on each patient—but as the information per patient grows in quantity, health care providers will need systems to help pull out subsets of data that are relevant to their particular subspecialties and to their unique ways of practicing medicine. Consequently, we find ourselves faced with the same dilemma that pervades other aspects of the information explosion in medicine: If we have more and more information available to us, we must find ways of making huge amounts of data manageable and accessible. Otherwise having so much information will be too much, and could prove as problematic as having no information at all!

Summary

This chapter provides the basic groundwork for understanding fundamental concepts in medical artificial intelligence. In addition to addressing the questions, "What is it?" and "How does it work?" the chapter raises issues about the benefits as well as the weaknesses of AI.

AI systems have been used primarily to assist health care providers to arrive at diagnostic decisions under conditions of uncertainty. Unfortunately, these systems are not as useful as they were hoped to be. While they can provide a useful "second opinion" of sorts, against which to evaluate one's own clinical reasoning and diagnostic conclusions, they are not sufficiently accurate to replace the reasoning of expert physicians. In fact, the best systems have been shown to perform about as well as first-year medical residents at the Massachusetts General Hospital.

On the other hand, research applications of neural network versions of AI have shown promise in uncovering patterns in the clinical courses of disease that permit predictions which surpass those permitted by more traditional prognostic models.

This suggests that AI might have more promise as a tool for analyzing research data than as an aid for bedside consultation.

On the horizon are AI applications that attempt to ensure more complete and accurate databases for each individual patient. While the notion of moving away from the problems of medical charts and human memory is certainly appealing, this change in information storage and retrieval can pose ethical dilemmas. As increasing amounts of information become available, questions will continue to arise regarding who "owns" the data, and how we will protect patients' rights in a world in which the computer card tells all.

Suggested References

Note: Most of the texts on AI that are appropriate to recommend for further reading were written in the mid- to late 1980s and the early 1990s. It may surprise the reader that such cutting-edge technology is not being discussed extensively in texts at the dawn of the new millennium. The likely reason for this is that the heyday of writing about AI in medicine occurred during the 1980s, because that was the time when scientists and computer programmers believed that AI systems would be the answer to many medical problems, such as the unavailability of subspecialty experts in some parts of the world. When AI proved to be less impressive than was hoped, much of the textbook writing dropped off. Current extensions of AI to medical practice may be seen at relevant professional conferences and in periodicals devoted to programming in this area.

Parsaye, K., & Chignell, M. (1988). *Expert systems for experts.* New York: John Wiley and Sons. This is a good place to begin to learn more about AI expert systems. It is geared to experts in a wide range of content areas and does not presume knowledge of computer programming. The book provides some information of historical interest and an excellent chapter titled, "A First Glance at Expert Systems." Additional topics that are well covered include dealing with uncertainty and the building of expert systems. There are excellent visuals to make the highly readable text even more user-friendly, yet it does not "talk down" to the experts who read it.

Buchanan, B. G., & Shortliffe, E. H. (Eds.). (1985). *Rule-based expert systems: The MYCIN experiments of the Stanford Heuristic Programming Project.* Reading, MA: Addison-Wesley. This book tells the story of the development of one of the first useful AI diagnostic systems, MYCIN. The project began in the1970s, and during the following decade resulted in a somewhat successful expert system for diagnosing infectious diseases. As the creators of MYCIN reflect back on their experiences, they also succeed in teaching a great deal about the process of building a successful expert system in a clearly defined area.

Weiss, S. M., & Kulikowski, C. A. (1991). *Computer systems that learn.* San Mateo, CA: Morgan Kaufmann Publishers. The authors of this book have an excellent track record in developing expert systems. Their goal for this book was to provide a text that would be useful in applied fields to help readers understand more about how expert systems "learn." The strengths of this book are two-fold: First, the emphasis on how systems learn leads the reader through an understanding of this phenomenon in a painless, thorough, and thoroughly interesting manner. Second, the book accomplishes something other texts have failed to achieve in an intelligible fashion: It forges conceptual linkages between AI methods and more traditional statistical approaches.

Citations in Text

Buchanan, B. G., & Shortliffe, E. H. (Eds.). (1984). (See Suggested References.)

de Groot, A. D. (1965). *Thought and choice in chess.* The Hague, Netherlands: Mouton.

de Groot, A. D. (1966). Perception and memory versus thought. In B. Klummintz (Ed.). *Problem solving.* New York: John Wiley and Sons.

Dreyfus, H. L. (1979). *What computers can't do: the limits of artificial intelligence,* revised ed. NY: Hayce & Row Publishers.

Evans, R. S., Pestotnik, S. L., Classen, D. C., Clemmer, T. P., Weaver, L. K., Orme, J. F., Lloyd, J. F., & Burke, J. P. (1998). A computer-assisted management program for antibiotics and other antiinfective agents. *N Eng J Med* 338(4): 232–238.

Feigenbaum, E. (1980). Knowledge engineering: The applied side of artificial intelligence. Memo HPP-80-21. Palo Alto, CA: Stanford University Artificial Intelligence Laboratory.

Lawrence, J. (1991). *Introduction to neural networks.* Grass Valley, CA: California Scientific Software.

Lindsay, R. K., Buchanan, B., Feigenbaum, E. A., & Lederberg, J. (1980). *Applications of artificial intelligence to chemistry: The DENDRAL project.* New York: McGraw-Hill.

Minsky, M. L. (1975). A framework for representing knowledge. In P. H. Winston (Ed.). *The psychology of computer vision.* New York: McGraw-Hill.

Montgomery, R. L., & Jordan, T. J. (1995). Predicting survival expectancy in HIV infected patients with pulmonary complications. *Proceedings of the second mathematical modeling conference: mathematical modeling for tuberculosis 1994.* San Francisco, CA: University of California.

Polanyi, M. (1972). *Personal knowledge.* Chicago, IL: University of Chicago Press.

Pople, H. E., Myers, J. D., & Miller, R. A. (1975). DIALOG INTERNIST: A model of diagnostic logic for internal medicine. *Proceedings of IJCAI, 75,* 849–855.

Shortliffe, E. H. (1976). *Computer-based medical consultation: MYCIN.* New York: Elsevier, North Holland.

Warner, H., Haug, B., Bouhaddou, O., et al., (1988). ILIAD as an expert consultant to teach differential diagnosis. In R. Greenes (Ed.). *Proceedings of the twelfth annual symposium on computer applications in medical care,* Washington, DC: IEEE.

Weiss, S. M., & Kulikowski, C. A. (1991). (See Suggested References.)

Index

Page numbers followed by f indicate figures; page numbers followed by t indicate tables.